Speak
Your Truth

*Proven Strategies for Effective
Nurse-Physician Communication*

Kathleen Bartholomew, RN, MN

+HCPro

Speak Your Truth: Proven Strategies for Effective Nurse-Physician Communication is published by HCPro, Inc.

HCPro, Inc., provides information resources for the healthcare industry.

HCPro, Inc., is not affiliated in any way with The Joint Commission, which owns the JCAHO and Joint Commission trademarks. MAGNET™, MAGNET RECOGNITION PROGRAM®, and ANCC MAGNET RECOGNITION® are trademarks of the American Nurses Credentialing Center (ANCC). The products and services of HCPro, Inc., and The Greeley Company are neither sponsored nor endorsed by the ANCC. The acronym MRP is not a trademark of HCPro or its parent corporation.

Kathleen Bartholomew, RN, MN, Author
Rebecca Hendren, Senior Managing Editor
Emily Sheahan, Group Publisher
Mike Mirabello, Senior Graphic Artist

Adam Carroll, Proofreader
Susan Darbyshire, Art Director
Jean St. Pierre, Director of Operations

Advice given is general. Readers should consult professional counsel for specific legal, ethical, or clinical questions. Arrangements can be made for quantity discounts. For more information, contact:

HCPro, Inc.
P.O. Box 1168
Marblehead, MA 01945
Telephone: 800/650-6787 or 781/639-1872
Fax: 781/639-2982
E-mail: *customerservice@hcpro.com*

Visit HCPro at its World Wide Web sites:
www.hcpro.com and *www.hcmarketplace.com*

05/2010
21768

Contents

Dedication ix

Acknowledgments x

About the Author xi

Foreword xiii

Introduction xv

Preface xix

Disclaimer-Acclaimer..xxi

Chapter 1: How It All Started: The Scope of the Problem 1

    What's the Problem?...6

    Big Problems...9

        Moral distress...9

        For your patients 10

        For your coworkers 10

        Burnout..11

        Work environment 12

Contents

Decreased job satisfaction 13

Retention... 14

Patient safety 15

Study at a Glance: Impact of Disruptive Behavior on Patient Care 16

Staffing levels 17

Factors Affecting Today's Nurses and Physicians 18

Physicians.. 18

Nurses 19

Conclusion.. 21

Chapter 2: Reasons for Poor Communication 27

Aha! Discovering Why We Can't Play Nice.. 29

The oppression theory 31

Power play 33

Sexuality as a mirror for power 33

Asserting their dominance 38

Tails between our legs 39

History: Why Jane Is Silent... 39

Game Over 41

Chapter 3: Key Stakeholders 45

Patients 45

What's our problem? 47

Physicians 47

Traditionalists and Baby Boomers..49

Generation X...49

The physician's point of view 50

Female physicians...51

Nurses..53

The agony 53

Powerlessness 54

The ecstasy..56

Caring..56

Boundaries 58

Adaptability 58

A healing environment...59

Nurse Managers...60

The manager's experience 61

Conclusion...63

Chapter 4: Checking the Emotional Pulse of Work Relationships....65

Part I: Taking the Pulse of Nurse-Physician Relationships...................66

Collegial relationships..67

Collaborative relationships...70

Teacher-student relationships...71

Friendly stranger relationships 72

Hostile relationships...73

Contents

Relationship Tips..75

Part II: Taking the Pulse of the Physicians 77

Part III: Taking Your Own Pulse 82

    No way 83

    Fear and uncertainty 83

    Maintaining our boundaries..86

    What would Jane do? 87

A Story of Courage and Confrontation 88

    What will Jane do?..88

Chapter 5: Breakdowns and Opportunities 93

Breakdowns in Communication 95

    Disagreements over discharge orders 95

    Disagreements over treatment decisions........................96

    Incidents of disruptive physician behavior....................97

    Telephone trouble...99

    The SBAR tool for preventing breakdowns..................100

Opportunities for Improvement..103

    Garner administrative support 103

    Create a zero-tolerance policy 104

    Provide assertiveness training 105

    Use your name as a powerful equalizer 106

Take advantage of formalized collaborative models 107

Build community 109

Strategies for Collaborative Relationships 111

Home runs! 111

Chapter 6: A Manager's Quest to Create Collegial Relationships... 117

The Power of a Name 118

Use Social Events as Networking Opportunities 122

The Great Fruit War: Conquering with Humor 123

Nursing Through a New Lens 123

A Meeting of the Minds 124

Creative strategies 126

Educational Opportunities 127

Just What the Doctor Ordered: A Physician's Prescription for
Transforming Our Culture 128

'Aunt Jane' 131

Setting the standard 133

Role modeling 136

Conclusion: Not So 'Pleasantville' 140

Chapter 7: Leadership's Role: Creating and Sustaining
Healthy Nurse-Physician Relationships 143

Perceptions vs. Reality 144

Individual Response: One Bad Apple 147

Contents

Process for Guiding Interventions 150

    Single unprofessional incident.. 152

    Apparent pattern of behavior 153

    Authority intervention 153

    Disciplinary intervention 154

System Response: ... Spoils the Whole Bunch.................................... 154

Start Here: Roadmap to Success.. 155

    Board and senior leadership commitment...................................... 155

    Set a standard of behavior/code of conduct 157

Code of Conduct: Education and Integration 157

    From theory to practice... 160

Create a Reporting or Surveillance Process 162

The Rest of the Bell Curve... 164

    Increase social capital.. 165

    Increase nurse educational level... 168

    Seek ANCC Magnet Recognition Program® status 169

    Conflict resolution skills 170

Hold the Vision.. 171

Nursing Continuing Education Instructional Guide 175

Dedication

I would like to dedicate this book to my parents, Dan and Alice Horneman. For my father who taught me how to write and my mother who taught me how to dream.

Acknowledgments

I would like to acknowledge that this book would not have been possible without the insightful and research-based contributions of doctors Alan Rosenstein, Gerald Hickson, Jon Burroughs, and Joe Bujak, as well as Debra Gerardi's work on conflict-competent organizations. I deeply appreciate their time, effort, and partnership on our journey to create collegial teams.

Thank you also to Nancy Loftin at Parrot Eyes Photography for the cover photo.

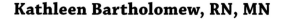

About the Author

Kathleen Bartholomew, RN, MN

Kathleen Bartholomew, RN, MN, managed a 57-bed orthopedic and spine unit in a tertiary hospital in Seattle for five years before turning to writing and public speaking full time. The first edition of *Speak Your Truth* was accepted as her master's thesis while studying at the University of Washington, Bothell.

As a registered nurse and counselor, Bartholomew uses story to bring to light the challenges and issues facing nurses today. Her strength is her ability to link the academic world with the practical reality of the hospital. Her objective is to serve as a much-needed voice for nursing today.

Bartholomew has been a national speaker for the nursing profession for the past seven years. Recognizing that the culture of an institution is critical to patient safety, she speaks about the image and future of nursing, creating healthy work environments, communication, nurse-to-nurse hostility, and improving physician-nurse relationships.

She is the author of the HCPro books *Ending Nurse-to-Nurse Hostility: Why Nurses Eat Their Young and Each Other* and *Stressed Out About Communication Skills,* and is the co-author of *The Image of Nursing: Perspectives on Shaping, Empowering, and Elevating the Nursing Profession.*

Foreword

This book is long overdue. If that statement seems hyperbolic, consider that even though nurses are an indispensable component of American healthcare, nursing as a profession is in crisis—due to the decreasing number of practicing nurses and the critical faculty shortage. Also, consider that in our post-IOM (Institute of Medicine) Report quest for increased patient safety, a nurse is a critical link in the processes that keep—or fail to keep—our patients safe from unnecessary harm.

So why do we need a book about physician-nurse relationships? Because for decades we have been working around and, in effect, hiding another truth: Poor relationships, poor communication, and compromised cooperation between physicians and nurses have a huge and frightening impact on our ability to keep patients safe from unnecessary harm and stay in a profession that too often demeans and devalues nurses.

This book is not an extensive complaint from the parochial perspective of an RN. Indeed, nurses not only respect physicians' central role in everything their profession accomplishes but also have a responsibility to create a renaissance in the way they and physicians work together. The closed-claim files of patient injuries are bursting at the seams with examples of disasters that resulted directly from ignoring the basics of teamwork.

Physicians who already understand in their gut and practice these methods of collegiality and teamwork will find this book an energizing validation. For those who have been trained to function in other ways, this work offers to show you, like Marley's ghost in

Dickens' *A Christmas Carol,* the unvarnished truth of the terrible damage that poor relations and poor communication can ultimately inflict on our patients and profession.

To say that American healthcare is evolving is a gross understatement. Medical technologies change by the day, and the advent of robust evidence-based medicine roars through the landscape of traditional medical training with a combination of promise and challenge. Coupled with the sudden discovery of how risky healthcare is from the patient's point of view, these changes have spurred us to reexamine everything we do—almost. We missed one thing, and covering it is the purpose of this book.

The traditional "design" of the nurse-physician relationship is worse than archaic in today's system; it is, quite simply, dangerous to life, limb, and profession. We must do more than lay this disturbing truth on the table—we must address it, and quickly.

John J. Nance, JD
A Founding Board Member of the National Patient Safety Foundation

Introduction

The Power of Culture

My first consulting engagement was to help a general surgeon who was about to lose his medical license due to his medical negligence regarding the deaths of two of his otherwise healthy post-operative patients who were both in their 40s. On both occasions, he performed a fairly routine procedure (Roux-en-Y bypass and a partial colectomy for diverticulitis) only to have both patients die because he refused to come into the hospital in the middle of the night to address post-operative complications (a leaking anastomosis for the Roux-en-Y bypass and an unaddressed bleeder for the partial colectomy that led to hypotension and an acute myocardial infarction). Why did he refuse a nurse's request to come in when in retrospect he knew that the nurse's request was based on sound judgment? He had an undiagnosed depression that paralyzed him and made it impossible for him to function late at night. What about the nurse? What was her role in these tragic events?

As it turned out, this general surgeon was not only considered the best surgeon on the medical staff but was also considered the best physician on the medical staff. He was compassionate, respectful of the nurses, collaborative, and extraordinarily dedicated to the healing arts profession. He graduated from a prestigious medical school and residency and was an innovative and dedicated healing force in the community, constantly pushing the envelope for bringing new services and technology to a relatively small and isolated healthcare environment. He was so good that his practice was enormous and he cared for thousands of patients who did not even need surgery; they just wanted a superb diagnostician and caring human being to minister to them and their families at their time of need.

Everyone on the nursing staff know that he had an undiagnosed depression. A dedicated family man, he had recently gone through a painful divorce because of his occasional outbursts of anger and abuse toward his wife. He would have rare outbursts on the medical floor and then the next day he would apologize for his disruptive behavior. The physicians and nurses covered for him out of respect, admiration, and a deep awareness of the magnitude of what he had brought to the community in balance. He was a beloved practitioner to all.

The two nights that his two post-operative patients began to fail, the nurse on duty covered for him by providing incremental measures at the bedside to address the patients' fever or hypotension because she did not want to "get the physician in trouble" or to expose what everyone knew was at the root of his pain. She knew that it was a violation of hospital policy and state law to not go up the chain of command in such an instance; yet, she admired and appreciated the physician not only because of his rare professional gifts, but because despite his undiagnosed issue, he always seemed to rise above his personal circumstances and to place the interests of his patients before his own. Unfortunately, by advocating for this wonderful physician, she abandoned her patients and partnered with the physician in inadvertently enabling them to die.

Sometime later, the physician took a leave of absence to get his depression treated and eventually returned to a successful practice, remarried, and made his peace with the devastation that his illness had caused. One day at a medical staff meeting, he asked the chief of staff why he and his colleagues had turned their back on him while he quietly suffered from a treatable illness. The chief of staff turned to him, looked him squarely in the eye, and simply stated, "I thought we were helping you by looking the other way."

Such is the nature of culture.

Culture is a powerful thing. It is not what we think, not what we say, not even what we intend; it is what we do at the end of each and every day. As Kathleen has poignantly and eloquently illustrated throughout the book, our culture is severely dysfunctional and broken. It is based upon a uniquely American myth that individuals are all-powerful and capable of professional perfection if they but work enough, sacrifice enough, and want it badly enough. Our culture is strewn with the broken lives of people and their families who have given everything to pursue this noble ideal, only to find they have over-reached, and in the process have damaged something deeper and even more precious: the right to be who we are and to accomplish in this life what we are really intended to do. The right to have meaningful work, rich and rewarding family lives, and passions that come from our heart and are often manifested through quirky hobbies, such as motorcycle riding, mountain climbing, or other pursuits, passions that seem to have no rational basis but provide some of the most important and meaningful experiences of our lives.

The traditional culture of the all-knowing and powerful physician with the deferential and self-abnegating nurse providing flawless medical and nursing care is a lie that must be systematically dismantled if healthcare is to remain important, relevant, and meaningful to those whom we serve. Unfortunately, it has been in existence, enabled, and supported for centuries and will not die an easy death. It must be carefully and sensitively taken down with deference and respect for what it has accomplished and with the urgency that recognizes the destructive impact that it has had on patients and on the medical and nursing staffs, both present and past.

We will need to rebuild a sense of meaning and mission to our shared work, awaken the growing realization that we are interdependent and rely on each other's knowledge and dedication to succeed in carrying out this important work, and realize that we cannot do it alone within the traditional self-imposed boundaries of our respective professions. Policies, procedures, tools, and best practices (e.g., SBAR) won't work until we dismantle the old culture and build something of greater value and sustainability in its place and create the policies and tools together.

Culture is not an abstraction or ideal, it is what we do alone and together when nobody else is watching or listening. It represents our true priorities and values and the decisions we make every day, both consciously or not. Physicians and nurses are both in pain today from the abuses of the past; however, we will never truly become a collaborative team until we are able to let go of our pain, release ourselves from this burden, and build something better together for ourselves, for the next generation of physicians and nurses, and for the patients whom we serve.

Jon Burroughs, MD, MBA, FACPE, CMSL
Senior Consultant
The Greeley Company

Preface

I feel lucky. I have numerous colleagues—physicians and nurses—from whom I receive a great deal of joy and satisfaction. It is empowering to know that I can call on a physician, and together we can resolve any situation. It is comforting to know that I can speak my truth, and the result will always be a clearer understanding and improved working relationships. There are many truly incredible physicians out there, and this book would do a great disservice if it did not recognize and applaud their contributions.

In fact, informal questioning reveals that less than 10% of physicians are disruptive or abusive. However, the effects are far greater. Perhaps it is simply human nature to allow a few bad apples to spoil the whole bunch. Nurses seem to recall negative relationships a lot more quickly than they can narrate the positive ones, which is why one of our challenges is to tell the good stories along with the bad. Although the focus of this book is on the damage caused by poor nurse-physician relationships, there are just as many stories that serve as tributes to the many physicians who work diligently every day to nurture partnerships, share their knowledge, and build collaborative relationships. These physicians set the standard for collegiality.

Remembering our code of ethics

E. Larson proposed in her article "The Impact of Physician-Nurse Interaction on Patient Care" that "failure of physicians and nurses to work together, to share decision making, and to communicate is not only undesirable, but is actually unethical because such behavior fails to focus on patient needs and can produce harm."

The Hippocratic Oath states that physicians should do good and not cause harm. In addition, the American Medical Association has adopted standards of conduct for professional physician behavior that state, "A physician shall uphold the standards of professionalism, be honest in all professional interactions, and strive to report physicians deficient in character or competence ..."

Likewise, the American Nursing Association code states that "the nurse is responsible for contributing to a moral environment that encourages respectful interactions with colleagues." This book demonstrates clearly that poor physician-nurse relationships cause harm. Is it ethical, then, to tolerate in any way a lack of collaboration and collegiality?

Kathleen Bartholomew, RN, MN

Disclaimer-Acclaimer

Disclaimer

To facilitate ease of reading, please note that pronouns used for physicians will be in the masculine form and those for nurses will be in the feminine form throughout the book.

Acclaimer

The names have only been changed to please my publisher, not to protect the innocent because, after all, nobody is innocent.

How It All Started: The Scope of the Problem

August 1992 ...

I was sitting at my desk fighting back tears when a concerned customer leaned over the telephone answering service counter. "What's the matter?" he asked kindly. I didn't need a mirror to know I looked awful. The night before, my husband had left for San Francisco. His parting words were, "You can come down later with the kids—if you want to." I didn't blame him. We had been arguing for more than two years, and arguing in San Francisco didn't seem like a much better option than arguing in Seattle. Still, emotion overwhelmed me when I realized that divorce was inevitable, that I was alone with five children under the age of 11, and that I was 3,000 miles away from my nearest relative. I started to explain all of this to Bob, who was a regular customer, when suddenly he took out his business card and scratched the name of a lawyer on the back. Then he wrote a check for fifty dollars and pushed it into my hand, insisting that I let him cover the first appointment. The very next week, my boss told me that I didn't have a job because the treasurer had embezzled the payroll and we were out of business. It was time to see the lawyer.

*   *   *   *

The early 1900s office building stood firmly in the heart of the city. Its dark, rich wood seemed to mimic the dreary Seattle weather, and the smell of mold in the elevator reminded me of a dank forest. I imagined myself effortlessly rising up a tree trunk as I climbed toward his office.

Inside, every chair, table, and desk was covered with books, papers, magazines, and overflowing cigar ashtrays. A thin layer of smoke hung two feet from the ceiling like a new-age mobile. My first thought was, "This was a mistake. My lawyer is Columbo." But within seconds, a portly gentleman was shaking my hand and laying out my worst fear, asking, "How are you going to take care of those five kids Bob said you have?"

"I don't know," I stammered, overwhelmed at the whole idea and wanting to vanish from reality like a genie into the safety of her judgment-proof bottle.

"Do you like nursing?"

"Well, my mother wanted me to be a nurse years ago, and I have always been interested in healthcare," I answered uneasily, taken aback by his candor. Then, hoping to score a few more points although uncertain of where the game was going, I added, "And I was a candy striper."

"I'll make you a deal," he said looking me squarely in the eye and reaching for his Bible. "I will do your entire divorce for $50 if you promise me that you will become a nurse." I barely needed time to think. I come from a long line of relatives who are proud of their thriftiness. Just last year, in fact, my sister was voted most frugal by my father when, after Christmas, she bought bags of M&Ms for 75% off the regular price and then had her children spend hours separating out the green for St. Patty's Day and the red for Valentine's Day.

I put my hand on the Bible. "Deal!" I said. I had bartered my divorce for my career.

*   *   *   *

Reality for me was always an afterthought—and this situation was no different. It hadn't occurred to me to consider the practical logistics of working, going to school, and raising five children, so when I applied to every school in Seattle and discovered there was a three-year waiting list, I was taken aback. I was 36. I didn't have three years. The only next step I could think of was to call my aunt, who taught nursing at her local university in North Carolina. She predicted that if I moved there, I'd be able to get into school within a year. It sounded like a good deal to me because just two weeks after I lost my job, a freak windstorm brought a hundred-foot pine tree crashing down on my house. When I cleared the branches from the entryway, I found a foreclosure notice stuck to the front door. Another message from the universe: time to leave town.

Camping across the United States with five children in a beat-up '76 Ford station wagon is a story in itself. Most nights, I'd lie half awake under the car, like a guard dog protecting my herd. When we finally arrived in Summerfield 10 days later, I was so exhausted that I slept for 17 hours.

We lived in a small trailer in the middle of 12 beautiful acres, adjacent to another hundred. My aunts helped watch the two youngest children until they were old enough for school. In order to finish my own schooling in two years, I had to take 22 credits a semester. Our car sat in the middle of a hay field, and after dinner, I would huddle inside it with a candle and my books so I could study in silence. Apparently, this was big news for a small town because the local paper ran a story about my incandescent habits.

Then one day, the nightmare was over. When they handed me my diploma, it was like receiving a gold medal. I couldn't stop crying from joy—and relief.

In my first nursing job, I was a medical-surgical nurse in a small community hospital. Orientation to the unit covered not only the skills I needed to care for the patients but also the knowledge I needed to survive working with the physicians. I was warned about the egotistical Dr. Keeting, to whom nurses were just another piece of furniture. When nurses spoke, he would glance only for a second in their direction, as if to say, "For a moment, I thought that chair said something." Then he would resume his charting without ever acknowledging that, indeed, the "furniture" had spoken.

It was also a well-known fact that if you called Dr. Keeting to notify him of a temperature of 103, he would hang up on you. I took care of his patients for weeks, and during this time his non-verbal communication made it clear that he expected me to be invisible. He would never make eye contact or acknowledge a mere nurse's existence—unless, of course, he had summoned her himself. As a new nurse walking into a culture that I didn't understand, I said nothing. I needed time to process this new environment, the strange interactions I saw between doctors and nurses, and my new clinical responsibilities.

Once I began to make sense of the situation, I couldn't believe the injustice that was occurring within the hospital. For the past two years, I had lived in a 500-square-foot trailer with five children, worked 30 hours a week, attended school full-time, and driven almost a hundred miles a day to work—so that I could be invisible? I don't think so.

One day Dr. Keeting decided he needed to speak to me. I had been waiting for this opportunity, like a panther in the grass, for weeks—not because I had anything planned, but because I knew that an interaction would not be meaningful unless he initiated it. At 6 ft. 4 inches tall, Dr. K. used his stature as yet another means of intimidation, so when he said, "I need to speak to you," I responded, "Just a minute." Then, to Dr. K.'s surprise, I pulled out the nearest chair, stood on it, looked him dead in the eye, and said, "How can I help you?" Stunned, he simply walked away. Within six months of graduating, I was promoted to charge nurse because of my ability to hold my own with the physicians.

In those first few years, I learned that the doctors' barks were worse than their bites. The next time Dr. Keeting came to the floor, I was less apprehensive. I mustered some courage and asked him if he had any children. Everyone was surprised when he stopped and took out his wallet to show us pictures of them—especially me. I had thought for certain that he would yell, "It's none of your business!" but he didn't. That simplest of human gestures seemed to shift the relationship.

With a few successes under my belt, I grew bolder and decided to see what I could do about one surgeon who intimidated the nurses with his order barking and brusque mannerisms. I found out that he was Irish, and the next time he came onto the unit, I softly began to hum "Sweet Rosie O'Grady," an Irish limerick taught to me during glee club in a convent basement as a child. After a few weeks of this, he lightened up so much that he even began singing to himself as he made his rounds. To this day, the manager talks about how I could get Dr. Sweeney to sing. These interactions taught me that simply connecting on a human level is an incredible catalyst for transforming physician-nurse relationships. It was a powerful lesson.

Of course, not all of my lessons were that easily won. After working for a few years in that small community hospital, I moved to a hospital that could have passed for a small city. My years there were a continuous challenge, and I only had one thing going for me: I stood up for myself. I didn't realize it at the time, but after two failed marriages, my "dukes" were up. I had been flattened twice in the boxing ring of life, and the fighting Irish in me wasn't going down a third time. I didn't know that it was the best thing I could do; all I knew was that every time I stood up for myself, I felt better.

What's the Problem?

I was reading at the bar in a local restaurant when the lady next to me leaned over to look at the title of my book. "Oh!" she said. "Are you a nurse, too?" Knowing that every nurse has a story, I asked for hers. "In 1983," she began, not needing even a second to recall a scene that happened so many years ago, "I was working in the AIDS unit of a teaching hospital in California when the resident asked me to start an IV. I simply couldn't because I was so busy. I was so far behind and had already started so many IVs. So I said, 'Why don't you?' He replied arrogantly, 'Because the patient has AIDS.'"

Every nurse I know can narrate at least one disturbing physician-nurse scene like this, and many of these stories have left deep scars. They are extremely personal and have been extremely hurtful to our pride, integrity, and profession.

It is no surprise that the most common feeling nurses experience after an incident of verbal abuse is anger (Araujo & Sofield, 1999). There is no healthy outlet for this anger, as it is seldom expressed except through horizontal violence, which is when powerless people lash out against each other. But this form of expression creates a new problem and fails to handle the primary emotion: hurt. And because the average age of nurses is now 48, many are carrying years of hurt in all they do. Therefore, even though a new generation of physicians is emerging, demographics prevent us from changing how we respond to them.

This problem has implications far beyond personal significance. Poor physician-nurse relationships affect morale, patient safety, job satisfaction, and retention (Larson, 1999; Rosenstein, 2002; Baggs et al., 1999). Such unhealthy relationships are hurtful to us and to our profession—and they aren't getting better. A survey published in the *Journal of Professional Nursing* showed that 90% of nurses had witnessed six to 12 unpleasant incidents between physicians and nurses within one year (Manderino, 1997). After reviewing the results of that survey, VHA West Coast—a division of VHA, Inc., a national network of community-owned hospitals and healthcare systems—surveyed 1,200 nurses, physicians, and executives (Rosenstein, 2002). Their results showed that 92.5% of respondents had witnessed disruptive behavior, which confirmed the findings of previous studies. One of the surprises of the VHA study, however, was that everyone defined the problem differently, identified different barriers, and proposed different solutions. All participants, however, agreed that poor physician-nurse relationships strongly affect morale (Rosenstein, 2002).

At the end of the VHA survey, an open-ended question asked respondents what could be done about the problem. More than 500 of the respondents suggested greater opportunities for communication and collaboration. So researchers began to study how communication and collaboration could enhance the physician-nurse relationship. In 1999, the SUPPORT care model was introduced. The Study to Understand Prognoses and Preferences for Outcomes and Risks of Treatments (SUPPORT) involved specially trained nurses who worked to improve care for more than 2,000 patients with similar ailments. The study structured a system of communication designed to change physician behavior by having nurses serve as important conduits of information (Larson, 1999). In this system, doctors had to go through the nurses to get information about their patients. The study tracked the outcomes in the following seven areas:

1. Patient-physician communication

2. Timing of do-not-resuscitate orders

3. Physician knowledge of patients' preferences regarding resuscitation

4. Number of days spent in ICU

5. Ventilation

6. Reported pain level

7. Hospital resources

But the study was a huge failure. The clinical trial resulted in no improvement in any of the outcomes. After two years of counseling and meetings designed to improve collaboration and communication, there was no improvement in physician-nurse relationships, and physicians still failed to hear what nurses said about their patients. Attempts to improve communication on its own failed.

The roles, interactions, and responses of the physician appear to have deep roots that even counseling cannot sever. And although the literature thus far has not been encouraging in terms of a solution, it has identified beyond doubt that there are serious problems that stem from poor physician-nurse relationships.

Big Problems

The stress that nurses manage is akin to being air traffic controllers—falling blood pressure in 42, crying patient in 44, irate doctor on the phone becoming impatient waiting for you (and you know it) as you struggle to help a patient to the bathroom. Nurses are extremely dedicated to their profession—even at the expense of their own time and health. We have a higher rate of "sickness presence" than any other profession—that is, coming to work even when sick to care for those sicker than ourselves. "The nurse is enculturated into an ideal that is derived from the nuns in religious orders who projected an abnegation of self in tender duty and obligation to others" (Sumner, 2003). But if we do not find our voice and do not recognize the forces that silence us, our profession will not survive.

Moral distress

I looked at the doctor's order three times, each time hoping that I had read it wrong. She had written the order quickly, totally ignoring me, and was obviously in a rush. My patient was dying. She was 90 years old and had stopped eating the week before in the nursing home. She had no family or friends. Chronic renal disease and a serious stroke had left her emaciated. As she lay motionless in the bed, she looked more like a withered plant than a human being. In my mind, she needed comfort care, but during rounds the doctor had written an order to insert an NG (nasogastric) tube and start supplementary feedings. Agh!

> *I went to the charge nurse, who pointed out that I needed to follow the doctor's order, but I couldn't do it. I tried to talk to the doctor, hoping to find some logic in the situation, but there wasn't a second where I could explain that there was no way I would ever treat my own mother like this. The doctor wouldn't listen. All I remember was her saying, "What's your problem again?" as if I were incompetent. It took me almost two hours to get up the nerve to call the chair of the Ethics Committee—and I did it from the lounge so the charge nurse wouldn't hear.*

For your patients

When nurses believe that one course of action is right for patients and physicians, who have the power to make the decision, either disagree or ignore nurses' positions, there is always moral distress: Nurses are forced to participate in a plan of care they believe is wrong. And without the final decision-making authority, we must stand by, powerless to change the situation. In this internal battle, the patient loses because such moral distress frequently leads to unfavorable outcomes.

For your coworkers

We live in a society that values cure over care, intellect over emotions, and science over art. Even though nursing is both an art and a science, society does not value it as such. So the pace of our daily lives continues to increase, regardless of how that affects patient care, and there is less time to connect with each other. This leaves us feeling alienated from our support system of many years. Today, in fact, we can only watch coworkers flounder instead of helping them because we too are "drowning" on the floor. This helpless feeling—this powerlessness and lack of autonomy—creates a great deal of moral distress.

In addition, as we spend less time with our patients in an effort to keep our heads above water, we are deprived of the joy of caring and connecting—the very reason we chose nursing in the first place.

Burnout

As a group, nurses lack power, and those who feel this lack of power struggle to be patient advocates in a system that does not reward advocacy (Sundin-Huard, 2001). This situation leaves us feeling paralyzed.

The current nursing infrastructure is modeled after the military, which uses the "chain of command" system. In this system, nurses must seek permission before taking any action, which robs us of our autonomy. In times of patient crises, however, it often proves to be useful: If we cannot get the answers or support we need, we can move up the chain of command. Start with your peers and the charge nurse, move on to the manager and nursing supervisor, and then, if necessary, speak to the physician on call or the department chair. If your concern is not validated, then at the very least, you and your peers will learn something new about the way your hospital functions.

If you stand by and watch a plan of care executed that is different than what you would advocate for a member of your own family, there is a high possibility that you are putting the patient at risk. Nurses are often put in this situation, and researchers have realized that such moral stress causes burnout, which causes nurses to leave the profession (Rosenstein, 2002; Corley, 1995).

> *At the end of the shift, the doctor stormed onto the floor looking for me. "Why did you call the Ethics Committee?" she said, glaring in anger. Loud enough so the charge nurse could hear, she hollered, "Why couldn't you just talk to me?" Right.*

Work environment

> *Nancy knew the physician was writing discharge orders for her patient because she had glanced over his shoulder to look in the chart. She approached him tentatively and said, "Doctor, your patient has a considerable amount of blood in his urine today." The doctor looked up at her annoyed and, with disgust in his voice, said, "So?" Later, he cancelled the discharge—without ever speaking to her.*

More than any other factor, the quality of relationships on a unit shapes the work environment. Studies show that improving the work environment is the best way to encourage nurses to remain in the profession. But to build significant and meaningful working relationships, we need time to do so, and to nurses and physicians, time is a luxury. Because of rising acuity, patient loads, decreasing reimbursements, and hospital cuts, health professionals must work harder and more quickly. Because healthcare is a business, there is a great deal of focus on profit and loss, but what we don't realize is that we have lost the greatest capital of all: social capital.

Social capital is the time we spend connecting with each other. Conversations about family, vacations, trials, and joys help create a feeling of belonging and community. When we share our lives, we connect through our humanity. We actively participate in creating an authentically caring environment where people are valued and appreciated. But in our fast-paced world, both physicians and nurses have started to view this time as trivial, soft, and unimportant, which negatively affects the workplace and job satisfaction.

Decreased job satisfaction

Lucía has been a nurse on the same orthopedic unit for 15 years, and her peers consider her an expert in her field. Lucía is pleased with the professional relationships she develops with patients because she knows that they feel safe and confident in her care. One day, a physician enters a room where Lucía is changing a hip dressing. In less than a minute, he berates and belittles her by questioning her competence as a nurse in front of the patient. Lucía is so embarrassed by the doctor's behavior that she walks out of the room.

In 2002, Dr. Linda Aiken of the University of Pennsylvania's Center for Health Outcomes and Policy Research released a study that made quite an impact not only on the healthcare community but on consumers as well. In her study, "Hospital Nurse Staffing and Patient Mortality, Nurse Burnout, and Job Dissatisfaction," Aiken found that higher emotional exhaustion and greater job dissatisfaction among nurses is strongly associated with higher patient-to-nurse ratios. Further, for every additional patient in a nurse's charge, there was a 23% increase in risk of burnout and a 15% increase in the risk of job dissatisfaction. Aiken stated that "40% of hospital nurses have burnout levels that exceed the norms for healthcare workers" (2002).

Another indication of poor job satisfaction is the fact that in 2001, 30% of new graduates under the age of 30 were planning to leave the profession within a year. A recent AMN Healthcare survey of 1,399 nurses found that almost half (44%) plan to make a career change over the next three years and more than one-third are dissatisfied with their jobs (AMN Healthcare, 2010). Clearly, dissatisfaction is increasing. The pace of work, level of stress, lack of meals and breaks, increased acuity of patients, and verbal abuse by physicians contribute significantly to an environment that provides little satisfaction or reward and is, at best, described as tolerable.

Retention

> *Rehema was in her fourth week of orientation on the unit when the charge nurse asked her to make rounds with the physicians. She proceeded to the first room, where the doctor was reviewing the chart just outside the door. She introduced herself and said the manager had asked her to round with the doctors so that she could become familiar with the physicians and learn from them. The doctor looked up for a moment, said nothing, and then continued going through the chart. Rehema waited patiently, and then followed him into the room. After several minutes of talking to the patient and ignoring her, he finally looked up and said, "Yes?" Rehema got the message. She gave up rounding with that physician and prayed that the manager would not expect her to try with another.*

According to an April 2001 study by the Federation of Nurses and Health Professionals, one out of five nurses now working is considering leaving the patient-care field for reasons other than retirement (2001). But what are the reasons? In a recent online survey (2001), 35% of participants said they left nursing specifically due to verbal abuse by a physician. These statistics are symptoms of a serious problem (Aiken, 2001).

Have you ever seen a domineering parent yell at a child, only to have the child turn around, run onto the playground, and push another child off a swing? This behavior is called "submissive-aggressive syndrome" and illustrates the simplest form of horizontal violence. Nurses do it all the time. The phrase "nurses eat their young" didn't come out of a fortune cookie. It came from observations we made to each other about our own culture.

Student nurses come onto the unit and (in a nursing shortage) we complain that they are in the way and they "just don't get it." But what they don't get is lunch—or dinner. And it's not okay with the new generation to go a week without a meal break.

We offer support to each others' faces, and yet talk behind each other's backs. This "don't rock the boat" style of communicating is common in nursing. As a profession, we have a passive-aggressive pattern of communication: We stay silent at times when we should speak, and speak up when we shouldn't. We complain to one another, but when a physician says something totally inappropriate, we are silent. While the boat may be still, we are taking on water.

Patient safety

Shanna thought she was immune to comments after 30 years of nursing. But still, the doctor's anger caught her off-guard. She felt certain that this patient had an ileus and it should be worked up immediately due to the patient's nausea and hypoactive bowel tones four days postop. Yet when she asked the physician for the tests, his tone was so angry and so vile that she fled to the bathroom, tears welling in her eyes. If he struck her it couldn't have hurt more.

When KLM flight 1422 crashed in March 1977, 583 people died. The world was shocked, and the airline industry reacted swiftly to determine what had happened. After listening to the cockpit recorder, investigators realized that the culture of the cockpit prevented the first and second officers from challenging the captain—and having done so could have prevented the crash. The airline industry took a hard look at the cause of this crash and others and developed a philosophy of "Crew Resource Management." In essence, it shifted the industry's culture from one in which the captain's actions were not to be questioned to one in which every member of the team was responsible to speak up when in doubt, to confirm and question orders, and to offer insight. It also made the commander take responsibility for creating and nurturing this type of environment.

Nine hundred twenty-three people die each week in healthcare settings across the United States as a result of medical mishaps. But because the bodies are scattered throughout the country, we don't see the terrible impact of such mistakes. If a Boeing 737 crashed every Monday, Wednesday, and Friday for an entire year, the number of deaths would be comparable to unnecessary deaths in healthcare (Leape, 1999).

In fact, the Institute of Medicine estimated in 1999 that 48,000–98,000 people die in the United States every year from medical errors. Five years later, in 2004, HealthGrades reanalyzed these numbers and concluded that not only were they accurate, but that they had been underestimated—and there have been no significant improvements in patient safety since the report's release. Preventable medical errors are now the third leading cause of death in America despite a call from the IHI and patient safety experts in 2006 to address the communication gaps which cause 84% of all sentinel events. And in a 2008 study, 77% witnessed disruptive behavior with physicians—which contributed to errors and death.

Study at a Glance: Impact of Disruptive Behavior on Patient Care

In a study of 102 hospitals with 4,530 participants (of which 2,846 were nurses) by the VHA West Coast:

- 77% reported witnessing disruptive behavior in physicians (88% RNs, 51% MDs)

- 65% reported witnessing disruptive behaviors in nurses (73% RNs, 48% MDs)

- 67% linked disruptive behavior with adverse events (medical error 71%, patient mortality 27%) (Rosenstein, O'Daniel, 2008)

Physician-nurse communication and collaboration are critical to patient safety (Baggs et al., 1999). An important study by Knaus, Wagner, Zimmerman, and Draper (1986), set in 13 ICUs, examined how staff interaction and coordination affected mortality. They were able to demonstrate that ICUs with positive nurse-physician relationships had a better risk-adjusted survival rate. They also found that communication and collaborative problem solving are key to patient safety, particularly for high-risk patients. Another study found that nurse-physician relationships are one of the seven categories of determinants of patient mortality (Tourangeau).

The Joint Commission instituted a National Patient Safety Goal in 2004–2005 that included "Improving the effectiveness of communication among caregivers." Nothing shapes the work environment more than the quality of relationships and communication styles on the unit. Improving physician-nurse relationships improves patient safety, but facilities still continued to tolerate bad behavior that affects patient care. In 2010, The Joint Commission required healthcare facilities to "establish a code of conduct that defines and sets out a process for handling unacceptable behavior."

Staffing levels

Significant research supports the claim that the nursing shortage and staffing levels greatly affect patient safety. A survey conducted by the Harvard School of Public Health and the William J. Kaiser Family Foundation, which was published in *The New England Journal of Medicine* (2002), found that 53% of physicians and 65% of the general public cited the shortage of nurses as a leading cause of medical errors. A study funded by the National Institute of Research found that every additional patient in an average hospital nurse's workload increased the risk of death in surgical patients by 7%. *Health Care at the Crossroads* (The Joint Commission, 2002) looked at 1,609 deaths and injuries since 1996 and found that low nursing staff levels were a contributing factor in 24% of the cases.

Dr. Linda Aiken concluded that "failure to retain nurses contributes to avoidable patient deaths." Nurses report greater job dissatisfaction and emotional exhaustion when they are responsible for too many patients (2002).

Factors Affecting Today's Nurses and Physicians

Physicians

> *When a fresh postoperative patient's blood pressure plummeted, I called the operating room to tell the surgeon that his patient's blood pressure had dropped to 78/40. I quickly organized my thoughts and relayed what I thought was the most important information. "She's not actively bleeding, and the reported blood loss in surgery was less than 200 cc." I was not prepared for his unmoved response: "Is that my third surgery today or my fourth?"*

Do you remember as a child seeing the car of a doctor with the caduceus symbol proudly displayed on the license plate? When was the last time you saw one of those? Television shows from the '70s and '80s typically portrayed the physician as an important and respected citizen. The symbol, the caduceus, used to guarantee that a physician could park just about anywhere and not get a ticket. Although it may seem like a small thing, it was a symbol of society's respect for the doctor. Back then, Good Samaritan laws were created to protect physicians from being sued when they stopped to help at an accident scene.

Recently, one doctor at our facility got a speeding ticket for going 80 mph as he transported a heart to another hospital. Even after he showed his identification and explained the situation, the policeman shrugged his shoulders and wrote the ticket. To the policeman, he was nobody special, and the heart in the cooler in the backseat wasn't a good enough reason to let him off the hook. After that incident, the doctor told me, "Times have changed."

Another factor affecting physicians is the sharp rise in malpractice insurance. Many physicians cannot afford to be in private practice any longer, so more are working for hospitals instead. Medical associations are advocating for tort reform in a society where consumers are "sue happy." Physicians are working longer hours for lower reimbursement rates.

Not only are physicians working longer, but they are working faster. "On average, a physician will interrupt a patient describing her symptoms within 18 seconds. In that short time, many doctors decide the likely diagnosis and best treatment" (Groopman).

In addition to these issues, "Doctors are unhappy about their loss of autonomy, falling income, and increasing workload," says LeTourneau (2004). Because of this loss of autonomy and ability to practice privately, physician assistants and nurse practitioners, whose positions were designed to help the physician, are often seen as threats. Under such circumstances, attempts at collaboration are thwarted because the physician perceives his coworkers as competition.

Nurses

"Take a break," said the charge nurse.

"I just can't," called back Julie. "They are calling for 964 for surgery NOW, and the second unit of blood is here for 68." It was 1:30 p.m. "I'll take a break after I get caught up," she said. The charge nurse proceeded to take the two new surgeries, and it was 4:00 p.m. before the two reconnected. "Missed meal, missed break" was written on both of their timecards—again.

Like physicians, nurses have also noticed an increased workload over the past few years, and because many nurses believe strongly in duty, obligation, and getting the job done, they are stretching themselves to the max. Patient acuity is higher and length of stay is shorter, which means that the patients who are in the hospital are sicker.

Also, due to the advances in medicine, hospitals are full of patients with chronic and secondary illnesses who in earlier years would not have survived. Advances in pharmacology have yielded a multitude of medicines, but with as many as 25 pills to give one patient, the stress level rises.

The nursing shortage has also resulted in an increased use of travelers and agency staff who fulfill important roles but who need to interrupt in order to ask questions because they are unfamiliar with the unit.

Because they are so busy, nurses have less time to spend with patients (e.g., one study found that patients receive less than 20 minutes of direct care in a 12-hour shift) and less time for interacting with the physicians (Ball, Weaver, & Abbott, 2003). This precious time spent interacting with each other builds relationships and supports nurses at work, but in the fast-paced healthcare environment, there is no time. Small talk is a luxury few can afford, so nurses miss out on the personal connections that produce job satisfaction and great working relationships.

It doesn't help that nurses are the least educated members of the healthcare team. More than half of the nurses in the United States do not have a four-year college degree. This disparity in education keeps the profession in the subordinate position—as the author of *Negotiating at an Uneven Table,* Phyllis Beck Kritek, says, we are playing at an "uneven table." Expecting a nurse with a two-year degree to communicate effectively and collaborate with a physician or pharmacist who has a doctorate is unrealistic.

> *There is no other profession that nurses must collaborate with professionally that does not require at least a four-year college degree. Given the wide disparity in education between nurses and other members of the healthcare team, clinical discussions that involve research, outcomes and clinical outcomes can be challenging at best (Knox & Simpson, 2004).*

Education is one of the most concrete actions that nurses can take to even the playing field. The push for evidence-based practice and standardization of care requires that nurses feel competent and knowledgeable in dialogue with physicians.

Conclusion

There is a severe nursing shortage. Nurses say the work environment is the most significant problem contributing to it, and nothing shapes the environment more than relationships. Now that poor physician-nurse relationships have been directly linked to higher patient mortality rates, administrators are paying more attention to the culture of relationships on the unit, but improving these relationships has proved to be a huge challenge.

What do we know about physician-nurse relationships? In a nutshell, research tells us that:

• Collaboration alone does not work

• Enhancing opportunities for collaboration does not work

- Units with positive physician-nurse relationships have decreased patient mortality rates

- Perceptions about the problem, barriers, and solution differ greatly between nurses, physicians, and administrators

- Empowering nurses and developing a positive role for them doesn't work because doing so doesn't alter the power structure, so nothing changes in the end

So where do we go from here? Both nurses and physicians need to understand how poor physician-nurse relationships started, recognize the forces that prevent us from having collegial relationships, and learn key practical strategies to change these relationships. As noted communication expert Susan Scott says, "Communication isn't about the relationship, IT IS THE RELATIONSHIP! If we don't feel free to comment or ask questions, then we don't have the collegial relationship with our physician partners that is so critical to patient safety."

In the end, improving communication with physicians is about creating an equal partnership where both parties respect and trust the roles each play in patient care. In a 2004 study, only 15% of physicians and nurses perceived that they had "excellent" relationships with each other, and only 25% were "very good" (Buerhaus, 2004). Clearly there is a tremendous opportunity to improve 75% of our working relationships. And because our relationships affect patient mortality, safety, retention, morale, and job satisfaction, improving our relationships is our ethical responsibility.

Elsie is the day charge nurse for the unit. The doctor approached the main station, like a soldier with a purpose, and said, "I need to talk to you. The patient in room 64 has an autovac and the blood was not reinfused." His voice grew louder. "What's the purpose of putting in the damn drain if you don't infuse the blood? I want a QI written out about this!" And before Elsie even has a chance to speak, he storms off the floor. "I'll look into it," she says to his back. "I'll look into it and get back to you," she says to the elevator doors as they close.

REFLECTIVE EXERCISE

Imprinting

Think back to nursing school. What was your very first interaction with a physician like? How did your early experiences as a student and new nurse shape how you deal with physicians today?

Does a story come to mind? Tell someone you trust your first RN-MD story.

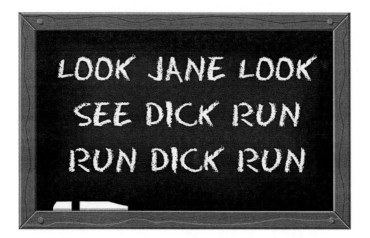

References

Aiken, Linda (2001). "Nurses' Reports on Hospital Care in Five Countries." *Health Affairs* 20 (3): 43–53.

Aiken, Linda (2002). "Hospital Nurse Staffing and Patient Mortality, Nurse Burnout, and Job Dissatisfaction." *The Journal of the American Medical Association* October 23/30.

AMN Healthcare. (2010). "2010 Survey of Registered Nurses: Job Satisfaction and Career Plans." *www.amnhealthcare.com/pdf/10_NurseSurveyWeb.pdf* (accessed March 9, 2010).

Araujo, Susan, and Laura Sofield (1999). "Verbal Abuse." *https://home.comcast.net/~laura08723/survey.htm* (accessed March 9, 2010).

Baggs, J.B., et al. (1999). Association Between Nurse-Physician Collaboration and Patient Outcomes in Three Intensive Care Units." *Critical Care Medicine* 27 (9): 2066–7.

Buerhaus, P., Donelan, K., Ulrich, B., Desroches, C., and Dittus, R. (2007). "Trends in the Experiences of Hospital-Employed Registered Nurses: Results from Three National Surveys." *Nursing Economic$* 25 (2): 69–79.

Corley, M.C (1995). "Moral Distress of Critical Care Nurses." *American Journal of Critical Care* 4 (4): 280–285.

Groopman, J. (2007). *How Doctors Think.* New York: Houghton Mifflin Company.

The Joint Commission (2002). "Health Care at the Crossroads: Strategies for Addressing the Evolving Nursing Crisis." *www.jointcommission.org/NR/rdonlyres/5C138711-ED76-4D6F-909F-B06E0309F36D/0/health_care_at_the_crossroads.pdf* (accessed March 9, 2010).

The Joint Commission. (2008). "Behaviors That Undermine a Culture of Safety." Sentinel Event Alert. *www.jointcommission.org/SentinelEvents/Sentineleventalert/sea_40.htm* (accessed March 15, 2010).

Knaus, W.A., P.P. Wagner, J.E. Zimmerman, and E.A. Draper (1986). "Variations in Mortality and Length of Stay in Intensive Care Units." *Annals of International Medicine* 103: 410–418.

Knox, E., and K. Simpson (2004). "Teamwork: The Fundamental Building Block of High Reliability Organizations and Patient Safety." Conference handout.

Kritek, P. (1994). *Negotiation at an Uneven Table.* San Francisco: Jossey-Bass Publishers.

Larson, E. (1999). "The Impact of Physician-Nurse Interaction on Patient Care." *Holistic Nursing Practice* 13 (2): 38–47.

Leape, Lucien (1999). *To Err is Human: Building a Safer Health Care System.* Cambridge, MA: Institute of Medicine.

LeTourneau, Barbara (2004). "Physicians and Nurses: Friends or Foes?" *Journal of Healthcare Management* 49 (1): 12–16.

Manderino, M.A., and N. Berkey (1997). "Verbal Abuse of Staff Nurses by Physicians." *Journal of Professional Nursing* 13 (1): 48–55.

Rosenstein, A. (2002). "Nurse-Physician Relationships: Impact on Nurse Satisfaction and Retention." *American Journal of Nursing* 102 (6): 26–34.

Rosenstein, A., and M. O'Daniel. (2008). "A Survey of the Impact of Disruptive Behaviors and Communication Defects on Patient Safety." *The Joint Commission Journal on Quality and Patient Safety* 34 (8): 464–71.

Sumner, J., and J. Townsend (2003). "Why Are Nurses Leaving?" *Nursing Administration Quarterly* 27 (2): 164–171.

Sundin-Huard, D. (2001). "Subject Positions Theory: Its Application to Understanding Collaboration (and Confrontation) in Critical Care." *Journal of Advanced Nursing* 34 (3): 376–382.

Tourangeau, A.E., L.A. Cranley, and L. Jeffs. (2006). "Impact of Nursing on Hospital Patient Mortality: A Focused Review and Related Policy Implications." *Quality & Safety in Health Care* 15 (1): 4–8.

Reasons for Poor Communication

For the next five years I worked as a staff nurse. During that time, I learned the art of dealing with physicians and quickly found that a sense of humor gave me more freedom to speak my mind. Once, when all the nurses were particularly frustrated with trying to decipher several doctors' handwriting, I used humor to address their concerns. I developed a game called "Guess That Order" for Nurses' Week. In it, teams of four nurses would have one minute to interpret a physician's hieroglyphics.

Simply walking around the unit to collect handwriting samples for the game was enough to get the point across. When I asked Dr. Nand what his orders meant, he looked hard at the paper and then after a few minutes said, "Get away from me. I am too busy for this." But I immediately called out to his back, "Oh my gosh! You don't know what it says either!" And as he turned away, I could see the traces of an ear-to-ear smile. I was right.

But even though I learned to use my sense of humor and read physicians' body language, I always took it personally when a physician became irate or was rude to me. It was the kind of hurt that cast a lingering shadow over the next few days—and I felt even worse when a fellow nurse was treated as if she didn't have a brain because it left me feeling helpless. My sense of humor alone could only get me so far.

Gloria came into the nurses' lounge, and I could tell by her contorted facial expression that something was wrong. "No doubt another hurtful interaction with Dr. Peters, judging from the dynamics earlier," I thought. She had gone directly to her locker and was blowing her nose as I searched for a way to make her feel better. "I guess Dr. Peters is in the doghouse," I said softly. No response.

Then I saw my inspiration in the trash—a brown paper bag. I grabbed a few markers, cut a doghouse shape out of the bag, and tacked it to the lounge bulletin board. I printed Dr. Peters' name on a piece of paper and boldly placed him in the doghouse. Not only did I get a kind of smug satisfaction out of this gesture, but when Gloria saw it, she smiled.

For months, the nurses would change the names featured in the doghouse according to the most abusive physician, and somehow it always made us feel better. But after six months, our secret was inadvertently discovered by a physician in search of birthday cake. Suddenly, he saw his partner's name in our doghouse and wanted to know why it was there. Then all of the doctors got curious and pried staff for additional information. After all, their egos were at stake. Doctors started to ask what scenes would send a doctor into the doghouse and would secretly peek through the door to make sure their names weren't up there.

> *The 3 West Doghouse, as it came to be known, succeeded in generating those much-needed conversations, which provided a means for nurses to state unacceptable physician behavior and gave physicians the opportunity to learn about their own behavior. One day, I heard our senior doctor cajole his junior partner, "I hope you're staying out of the doghouse?" It was a gradual change, but over the course of the year, the atmosphere on the floor became much more casual due to our doghouse, which had allowed staff a means to speak their truth.*

Then, one day, my entire perspective shifted. I enrolled in a master's of nursing program. One of my assignments was to write a term paper about physician-nurse relationships, and the more I learned, the less I took confrontations with physicians as a personal assault. Everything made perfect sense. For the first time, I could see the role that nursing played in keeping the physician-nurse game in motion.

Aha! Discovering Why We Can't Play Nice

Unless we understand nurse and physician behaviors, we will never significantly improve physician-nurse relationships. That's why attempts at teaching physicians to collaborate and nurses to communicate have failed up to this point—neither party truly understands the power dynamics between them. Past attempts at improving physician-nurse relationships have also failed because nurses refuse to acknowledge just how personally we take physicians' verbal assaults and intimidation tactics. Instead, nurses downplay the effects of poor relationships by rationalizing them away and saying, "It's just part of the job," or by acting on the belief that we can handle any situation. But the fact of the matter is that **you cannot ignore a wound and fix it at the same time.**

Just as in nursing school, where we were taught to inspect the wound and assess the damage, diagnosing and assessing the damage caused by poor physician-nurse relationships is necessary for healing. The first step is to identify the game. Second, we must understand why we keep playing it. Third, we must learn key strategies to put it to an end. The best way to follow these steps is to look at history and theory. History tells us where the problem started and how it took shape. Theory helps us understand the forces that keep the problem in motion. So history tells us why Jane is so silent, and theory tells us why Dick runs and roars.

Power can be subtle and illusive. For instance, I have an acquaintance who has her PhD in nursing. Her colleague is a physician, and together they travel throughout the country teaching about quality and safety in healthcare. After a short time, she noticed that her name was always second on the billing and that the physician was introduced as "doctor" while she was always introduced by name. When she pointed out this inequity, he said, "Just get over it."

When someone tells you to "get over it," it's because he or she doesn't understand what "it" signifies to you. And from his position, the physician could see no problem, but that's not how the nurse saw it. After 10 years of programming as a result of climbing the educational ladder, the doctor's view was clearly different. It's as if the physician was viewing reality from an entirely different plane—from a plane that didn't allow him to understand his colleague's perspective. Research consistently shows that physicians and nurses have such differing views not only about problems but also about the barriers and solutions surrounding them (Rosenstein, 2002).

One significant factor behind these differing views is that physicians go through medical school and nurses do not. Studies show that every year of medical school produces a medical student who is less empathetic than the year before (Thernstrom, 2004), which should come as no surprise. Think about it. Residents often work 80–100 hours in a single week, and their energy is stretched to the limit. They also face highly emotional situations at a breakneck pace. In order to function under such tremendous pressure, residents must rely heavily on logic. Their minds are trained to compute like an algorithm chart for Advanced Cardiac Life Support, and in order to process the sheer volume of such work, the flow chart for emotions is deleted.

Lacking the luxury of time, they are unable to process or digest the intense emotions (e.g., grief, death, and loss) associated with their work. And so, with the cold logic of computers, residents must rewire, or adapt, to survive. They create work-arounds, deleting feelings in order to focus on the task at hand.

Columbia University is attempting to address the issue of decreased empathy by requiring all second-year residents to take a seminar in narrative medicine (Thernstrom, 2004). The goal is to help medical students process and express emotions that were previously ignored. In this way, the paradigm is shifting, but again, the average age of a nurse is 48; many of us still carry wounds of the past and continue to take physicians' negative behaviors personally.

The oppression theory

The existence of unequal relationships—such as those between high-income and low-income, white and non-white, men and women—can be explained by perceived or actual differences in power. In his book, *Pedagogy of the Oppressed*, Paulo Feire studies the dynamics of these relationships in-depth. He explains that whenever there is a dominant and a subordinate group—whenever there are two groups and one has more power than the other—oppression occurs. This is called the oppression theory. The interesting part about the theory is that both groups agree to the rules of this unequal game and continue to play it. It is not only the dominant group that makes the rules, but the subordinate group that reinforces them by adhering to them.

Oppression theory fits medicine like a glove. Twenty years ago, when the physician arrived on the floor, both parties expected the nurse to stand up, give her chair to the doctor, and scamper off to bring him a cup of coffee and a donut. This behavior was not written anywhere, but it was generally accepted and widely practiced. This power play still exists today, but it has become more subtle. When the physician arrives on the floor, for instance, the nurse immediately hands him the chart, even though she has not finished writing her entry. When a nurse calls the physician after hours, the conversation often begins with "I'm sorry to bother you ... ," as the nurse unconsciously puts herself into the subordinate position. Questions about patient care are answered abruptly, with poor eye contact from both sides.

The complete absence of a relationship between the two parties is a result of this power game. This is why, when a nurse walks into a room, the physician will look up from his chart and ask, "Do you need something?" as if she were an unwelcome intruder instead of a valuable team member whose knowledge and assessment he depends on for quality care.

The problem here is two-fold: Expectations are set by dominant physicians and are held in motion by nurses who continue to perform them. There are two main forces that keep this game in motion: 1) we are not aware of the power play, and 2) historically, we have not had a voice. In the book *From Silence to Voice,* two journalists struggle to understand why nursing has so little presence in the media. They were surprised to discover just how embedded silence is in our profession—if we can find our individual and collective voices, we will reclaim our power.

Power play

Power can be used to enhance, control, or destroy a relationship. A powerful relationship can be fulfilling for both parties or make life miserable for those involved. Power is what makes collaboration such a challenge. Because collaboration requires a balance of power, some physicians view it as a threat to their autonomy. In these cases, collaboration becomes synonymous with insubordination and is perceived as an erosion of physician power.

As nurses, we are immersed in a culture of relationships based on power. The relationships of doctors and nurses have for centuries paralleled the relationships between men and women in our society. And because power is often subtle and so embedded in the physician-nurse culture, it is often difficult for us to recognize.

Sexuality as a mirror for power

Trying to discuss power is like a fish trying to describe water; we are so immersed in the subtleties that it is impossible to see their effects. In fact, one of the key characteristics of oppression is that the rules of behavior are so ingrained in the culture that no one acknowledges them. A power play that is more obvious has a better chance of clarifying the oppression theory, so we will review one that is fairly universal: sexuality.

The dynamics of sex work beautifully to explain those inherent in physician-nurse relationships. Like power, sex can help a relationship blossom and deepen with the result of two people feeling energized by each other's presence, or it can demoralize and destroy a relationship until both people are limp and frigid.

The limp and frigid theory

The frigid nurse

The frigid nurse cannot express herself intellectually. When she calls the attending physician to report a low potassium level of 2.5, the nurse hears him say, "So what do you want me to do about it?" and shuts off completely. She knows quite well what she wants him to do, but once upon a time, in an idealistic world far, far from reality, she offered her opinion and the doctor belittled her—so now she refuses to put herself in that vulnerable situation again. In a nanosecond, her body and mind have tallied every lousy interaction she has ever had with a physician, and the vote is in: It's not worth it. She says nothing.

Even the very question "So what do you want me to do about it?" is intimidating. But as a woman who is twice divorced, has five small children, and has scratched her way out of a hole to become a nurse, she might say something she'll later regret, such as:

> "I want you to pick a letter, doc:
> a)   Do nothing
> b)   Redraw the lab value and check the diuretics this patient is on
> c)   Do nothing
> d)   Both a and c"

Demonstrating intelligence and using your voice are characteristics of the dominant group, not the subordinate group to which nurses are supposed to belong. As in any other relationship, the role that we have been socialized into and the role that we have rehearsed prevents us from being our amazing selves. Weak responses, lack of action, and avoidance behaviors keep nurses in this subordinate position, but we must realize that these are learned behaviors that have been shaped by centuries of cultural reinforcement.

Awareness of this cultural oppression is the catalyst for change (Feire, 1971). What if nurses stopped playing by these unspoken rules? What if, when we were working on a chart, we didn't automatically hand it to the newly arrived doctor unless he asked for it? What if we made the bold assumption that nurses and physicians are peers? What if we held the vision for a collegial relationship, asked questions, and focused on our common humanity?

The latter is one of the most powerful ways to even the playing field. Talk to a physician about a subject that has nothing to do with work. For example, if you discover something as simple as the fact that you and a physician have kids on the same soccer team, your relationship will never be the same. You are no longer just his idea of a nurse—you are a person with a name—and that automatically shifts the energy of the relationship.

The limp doctor

The limp doctor cannot express himself humanely. He does not want his position as omnipotent physician to be challenged—if it is, staff might see him as a mere human being. But he must uphold the power difference at all costs because years of education and socialization have taught him how a doctor is to act—superior. Keenly aware of the boundary between the professional and personal, he will go out of his way to remain professional at all times—but his Achilles' heel is his humanity.

The aloof, businesslike stance is mandatory to maintain the dominant position. Any questioning of authority is rebuffed to protect the position of power, which is why he cannot possibly address the nurse as a partner. Indeed, one of the most common ways he negates the nurse with whom he works is by never learning her name. If he cannot protect this dominant position in this way, he will go limp.

Casey calls the hospitalist because her patient is experiencing a severe exacerbation of chronic obstructive pulmonary disease (COPD). Despite her report that the patient's oxygen is increased to 8L and that he is breathing 36–40 per minute with difficulty, the hospitalist downplays the problem and does not come to the floor. An hour later, Casey calls the doctor again and insists that he see this patient right away. He says he will come when he can, completely ignoring the urgency in her voice.

Having gotten nowhere, Casey calls the manager, who calls the hospitalist. The hospitalist says, "The patient's blood gases were fine this morning," but that he will go and see the patient at her request. "What do you want me to do?" he says defensively when he gets to the floor.

Casey has a plan. She says, "I want you to order some IV Solumedrol to open up this poor patient's airways so he can breathe more easily." Now, because the hospitalist will take Casey's suggestion, he cannot keep up the appearance of superiority—in other words, he goes limp. To assert himself, he pulls out all the tricks of the trade. His voice becomes louder and his body language turns angry. He writes orders for the IV drugs and transfers the patient to the transitory care unit, saying, "If you nurses on an orthopedic floor can't take care of a simple COPD exacerbation, then I will transfer this patient to a floor with competent nurses who can!" The next time he is seen on the unit, he ignores everyone, and the nurses who are still hurt by his comment ignore him because they want to avoid another scene.

All physician actions, comments, and non-verbal communications are designed to keep them in the dominant position. This stems from a time when nurses' treatment was more akin to that of indentured servants than to that of healthcare professionals. For example, some physicians of the early 1900s claimed that nurses did not need an education because the physician was already educated: "In 1908, William Alexander

Dorland ... delivered his graduating address urging nurses to accept the importance of their intellectual inferiority ... and warned that nurses should never aspire to such heights; for them to do so was not only 'dangerous,' it could be 'fatal' " (Ashley, 1976, 77).

And there we have nursing's "fatal attraction": Critically think and die. This message has been passed down through the generations, and it is evident in nursing practice today.

Nancy works in a renal transplant unit. She is considered an expert in her field and could run operations single-handedly. Yet the doctor turned to her yesterday and said condescendingly, "Nancy, now you know better than that." What Nancy knew was that she needed a physician's order for blood prior to a procedure. So she had the resident call the physician, only to have the doctor turn the situation around to make her look incompetent.

It would be naïve to think that physicians learn only medicine in medical school. Rather, physicians learn a multitude of rules about how to interact with other members of the healthcare team. The medical educational system is perfectly designed to ingrain these behaviors into the graduating doctor's personality. Residency was actually "Role Modeling 101," where the physician learned all the tricks of the trade—all the ways to keep nurses in the subordinate position. One of my favorite such tricks is the single-word answer: "And?" "So?" "Yes?"—all said with just the right amount of caustic sarcasm. For such educated people, physicians use a lot of one-word sentences.

Like animals

Humans often mirror animals. And as such, men have developed a set of universal behaviors to demonstrate their believed superiority. In fact, the members of any cultural group, whether male or female, learn a set of behaviors characteristic of their group. Sociologists call this process "enculturation." Although the behavior is not taught formally, younger people learn it by watching the actions of older people. And the behavior often continues for generations because of positive reinforcement. The same pattern of learning holds true within healthcare.

Asserting their dominance

Physicians have a unique and subtle set of behaviors designed to keep them in the dominant position. But it's important to recognize them for what they are—learned behaviors. If we forget this, we will take arrogant and rude behavior personally and be wounded by it. We will assume that the behavior is directed at us, but the truth is that these learned behaviors are a part of the physician culture. The most obvious of the learned behaviors is tone of voice. You will likely hear it in the tone that delivers the intended message, "You are bothering me."

In the healthcare culture, doctors often use intimidation and aloofness to control. For example, little or no eye contact is designed to deliver the message, "You are not even important enough for me to acknowledge your existence." Similarly, a deep and short tone shows annoyance and is meant to leave the nurse saying ridiculous things such as, "I'm sorry to bother you, but ..." every time she calls.

Another example is in the operating room. There, physicians literally expand their chests and put their arms stiffly and deliberately through their gown in an "I am a surgeon!" gesture. Healthcare, like any realm, has its own set of norms.

Tails between our legs

Nurses also have their set of learned behaviors, both from school and from orientation to the hospital setting. Typical nurse behaviors mentioned earlier include apologizing for a phone call and automatically handing a doctor the chart, but the most noticeable are avoidance behaviors. Nurses will literally duck into rooms when a physician they don't like comes down the hall—or if they see a doctor with whom they have had an unpleasant interaction in the past decade.

In addition, nurses often demonstrate poor or nonexistent communication skills. Freedom to ask questions of the doctors with whom we work is restricted because, from experience, we know which doctors will be—to put it nicely—unreceptive. So we don't ask and we don't learn, which keeps us ignorant—and ignorance keeps us in the subordinate position. This is the doctor-nurse game. As the old saying goes, "Knowledge is power." Some doctors actively prevent nurses from understanding their plan of care because obstructing nurses' knowledge allows doctors to hold onto power. Why do nurses put up with this behavior?

Because according to the rules, if Jane speaks her truth, the game is over.

History: Why Jane Is Silent

The domestic origins of nursing are one of several factors affecting the profession today. Nursing originated in a culture where men were viewed as superior to women. In this patriarchal world, the primary role of women was that of a domestic helper who needed supervision, but in the 1900s, nurses experienced autonomy in the home setting, especially in their roles as midwives. Then, when healthcare was institutionalized, nursing practice came under the direct control of physicians. Nurses were educated in physician-run hospitals, which further served to enforce their subservient role. This setting allowed physicians to assume the role of teacher, which gave them total power over curriculum decisions (Ashley, 1976).

Another factor is that, historically, caring was the nurse's primary role. It was viewed as "a woman's duty to [her] family and community" (Reverby, 1987). This original belief system continues to cause problems today because society ostensibly does not place value on caring.

Still another part of the problem is the Western medical model of separation, dissection, and objective thinking, and its heavy influence on medicine. This model favors curing over caring and devalues the nursing profession as it was established by Florence Nightingale in the late 1800s. Nightingale established caring as a key component of the nurse's roles, but physicians taught the Western medical model, which championed objective and linear thinking, not the subjective, holistic approach and art of caring that was intrinsic to early nursing. Rather than allow both models of healing to complement each other, nursing was molded into the medical model that did not value or acknowledge nursing's unique contribution.

Although the role of women has shifted over the generations, we still live in a male-dominated society (Faludi, 1992). Therefore, gender imbalance also comes into play. Due to the large number of females attracted to nursing—and its domestic origins—the profession was stereotyped as a woman's job (to this day, 85% of the healthcare work-force is female). The deep-rooted assumptions about gender continue to polarize physi-cian-nurse relationships, as illustrated in the following quote by Jo Ann Ashley, an expert on sexism in nursing:

Modern nursing originated at a time when Victorian ideas dictated that the role of women was to serve men's needs and convenience. Nursing's development continued to be greatly influenced by the attitudes that women were less independent, less capable of initiative, and less creative than men and thus needed masculine guidance (Ashley, 1976).

Physicians operated from this perspective for other reasons as well. Economically, the nurse has always been a potential threat to the medical field because her knowledge and legal recognition of her competence threaten the physician's position of authority (Ashley, 1976). The fact that nurses came mainly from the middle class and physicians from the upper class is another significant contributor to the inequity. This difference in socioeconomic standing reinforced the idea that physicians were better than nurses because they came from a higher class background.

From a historical perspective, therefore, the subordinate role of the nurse has its roots in gender distinctions, the origins of the professions, and socioeconomic status (Larson, 1999). This unequal power footing is the root of all discord in physician-nurse relationships. Add to the problem the vast gap in nurses' education and it's clear why Jane is silent: She never thought she had a chance.

Game Over

The dynamics between nurses and doctors have been studied since the late 1960s by Leonard Stein (1987), who first described the behaviors that are now referred to as the doctor-nurse game. Stein noted that nurses asked questions in a manner that preserved the physician's ego by presenting concerns and information as if they were the doctor's idea. For example, the doctor has written orders and is leaving the floor. The nurse picks up the chart and notices that he did not order any labs despite a hematocrit of 27 on her patient yesterday. She says, "Excuse me, did you want to order any labs today?" This jars the doctor's memory so that he says, "Why yes, I did." No, *he* didn't. Game on.

Coming from an equal power footing, however, the nurse would have said, "I noticed (yes, I noticed! *Me! Me! ME!*) that Mr. Smith's hematocrit was 27 yesterday—I think we should repeat the HCT?" What a big difference!

To avoid playing the game, we must constantly be aware of when we give away our power. Doing so takes a constant vigilance and honesty with oneself. I know all of this, and even I played the doctor-nurse game just recently. The patient coded in room 961 from presumably pulmonary edema, and 40 cc of Lasix had already been given intravenously. I seemed to be the only one who noticed that the IV was still infusing at 150 cc, but because I didn't know the physician, I said, "Did you want to change the IV rate?" to call his attention to the fluids, instead of saying, "The IV is running at 150. I am turning it down to 40." I could have kicked myself.

Every time a physician is intimidating, and every time there is verbal abuse and the nurse says nothing, we keep the game in motion. Herein lies the key to change: What if nurses no longer played by these unspoken rules?

> *Barb had a reputation for being the best at arterial line management in the ICU. One day when she was busy, the physician asked a new nurse to help him with the line. She said, "I'll find Barb." The physician responded loudly, "Any well-trained baboon can manage an art line." From behind the curtain in another room, Barb had heard the entire conversation.*

> *A week later, the same physician again asked for assistance with an art line, but this time the nurse's response surprised him. Barb shouted from the clean supply, "Just find a well-trained baboon!" It took the physician a minute to remember, but he got the message.*

       Speak Your Truth

R E F L E C T I V E   E X E R C I S E

Take Two

Think back to your last uncomfortable interaction with a physician. Scan the scene as if you were observing yourself in a TV show. Did you unconsciously put yourself in a subordinate position using comments, body language, or tone of voice?

Think back to your last collegial interaction with a physician. How was your response different? What language or body language did you demonstrate that indicated you stayed "in your power"? How did you feel in this interaction?

Focus on what it feels like to be "in your power" and try to keep this feeling in every interaction.

References

Ashley, J.A. (1976). *Hospitals, Paternalism, and the Role of the Nurse*. New York: Teachers College.

Buresh, Bernice, and Suzanne Gordon. (2000). *From Silence to Voice: What Nurses Know and Must Communicate to the Public*. Ithaca, NY: ILR Press.

Faludi, Susan (1992). *Backlash: The Undeclared War Against American Women*. New York: Anchor Books, Doubleday.

Feire, P. (1971). *Pedagogy of the Oppressed*. New York: Herder and Herder.

Kramer, M., and C. Schmalenberg (2003). "Securing 'Good' Nurse/Physician Relationships." *Nursing Management* 34 (7): 34–38.

Larson, E. (1999). "The Impact of Physician-Nurse Interaction on Patient Care." *Holistic Nursing Practice* 13 (2): 38–47.

Reverby, Susan. (1987). *Ordered to Care: The Dilemma of American Nursing, 1850–1945*. Cambridge: Cambridge University Press.

Roberts, S. (1983). "Oppressed Group Behavior: Implications for Nursing." *Advances In Nursing Science* 5 (4): 21–30.

Rosenstein, A. (2002). "Nurse-Physician Relationships: Impact on Nurse Satisfaction and Retention." *American Journal of Nursing* 102 (6): 26–34.

Stein, Leonard I. (1987). "The Doctor-Nurse Game." In *Dominant Issues in Medical Sociology, 2nd edition*. New York: Random House.

Thernstrom, M. (2004). "The Writing Cure: Can Understanding Narrative Medicine Make You a Better Doctor?" *New York Times* (4): 45.

 Speak Your Truth

3

Key Stakeholders

In order to improve nurse-physician relationships significantly, we must understand the barriers, power struggles, and roles of the key stakeholders: patients, physicians, nurses, and nurse managers. Because none of the key stakeholders can remain unaffected by the actions of the others, it is critical to understand the nature of these relationships. As Einstein said, "The belief in our separateness is an optical delusion." What effects do our behaviors have on each other?

Patients

Mr. Wagner was in serious pain. "Can't you do something?" begged Mrs. Wagner, who had spent the night with her husband and was visibly upset.

"No," the nurse responded firmly, but with sympathy. "I've already given your husband the highest dose of medication possible without having to worry about side effects."

> *"Can't you call the doctor?" Mrs. Wagner pleaded.*
>
> *"No," said Julie. "The doctor has already left specific pain orders." The truth was, however, that the last time Julie had called Dr. Martin after hours, he had yelled at her. She was desperately trying to postpone calling him until "a reasonable hour." It was 4 a.m., and if she could just manage the situation until 7 a.m., Dr. Martin would be much more amicable.*

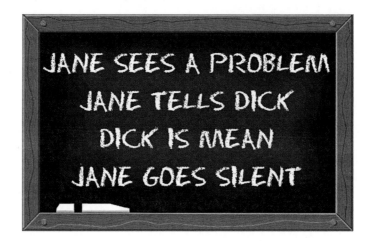

The *patient* pays when Dick and Jane can't get along.

Too many physician-nurse interactions follow the above formula, and when physicians and nurses have such negative interactions, communication suffers, and it's the patient who loses. In such situations, the problem is ignored or not addressed in a professional manner, which ultimately results in poor working relationships and negative patient outcomes.

Poor communication is the primary cause of patient error. Of 2,455 sentinel events analyzed by The Joint Commission, 70% of the cases were due to communication failure. How serious were these communication errors? According to The Joint Commission, 75% of the involved patients died. "We can create an environment in which individuals can speak up and express concerns" (Leonard, Graham, & Bonacum, 2004), and in such an environment we can catch and correct each other's mistakes instead of watching helplessly as they occur.

What's our problem?

Within the healthcare system, we have set up for ourselves the unattainable goal of perfection. Under this goal, we often neglect to question each other and, in turn, prevent ourselves from communicating effectively. We, therefore, can improve communication by dispelling myths that say "a good nurse/physician does not make mistakes" and "practice makes perfect." If instead, we accept our humanity, focus on the strength that comes from community, and build solid relationships, we can create an environment that supports all stakeholders in a realistic manner. In addition to finding our voice, what we say must be acknowledged, respected, and acted upon. Until that happens, negative outcomes will continue to occur.

Physicians

What could possibly trigger the physician behavior that shuts nurses down?

Ego boosting to do the job: A brain surgeon once told me that it takes a big ego for him to perform some operations, and that if he didn't nurture his ego, he'd wonder sometimes whether he could even perform them.

High expectations: Physicians are expected to have all the answers, so when they don't, sometimes they snap. Mistakes are viewed as incompetence, and perfection is expected.

HMOs: Many doctors work for large health maintenance organizations (HMO) that dictate, for example, strict lengths of stay. Finances alone put additional pressures on all physicians.

Sheer pressure: Falling reimbursement rates and rising malpractice costs both dictate longer working hours. Add to this patient overload, loss of autonomy, bureaucratic red tape, and technology, and it becomes increasingly clear why stress has increased for physicians (Bujak, 2008).

> *As I walked into the hospital on Saturday, the loudspeaker boomed with a sense of urgency that even a visitor could not ignore: "Will ANY senior-year surgical resident please call 3000 stat?" Three times the announcer's voice called out, as if he were watching a patient crash before his very own eyes. I sighed with relief that I was not that resident. What pressure!*

More important than all of the above issues, however, is physicians' recent loss of autonomy and prestige. A cartoon in *The New Yorker* magazine summed it up. In it, a mother and daughter hovered in the doorway while a little boy with a doctor's kit stood on the sidewalk. In the caption, the girl said to the boy, "My mother says I can't play with you unless you pretend to be something else." Another sign of the physician's declining public importance was recently illustrated on the cover of *U.S. News and World Report*, which read: WHO NEEDS DOCTORS?

Understanding where physicians are 'coming from' is very helpful. In his book, *Inside the Physician Mind*, Joe Bujak, MD, describes this culture, noting that autonomy is the core value of the profession.

> *Physicians are a result of their training, which is hierarchical. Physicians progress through training as one would ascend the rungs of a ladder. In this setting, it becomes culturally difficult to accept input from the people perceived as being below you. They are highly competitive and predisposed not to trust. Because of their sense of omniscience and omnipotence they are quick to interrupt and draw conclusions. In addition, physicians are trained to approach problem solving by deductive and linear reasoning which is in contrast to the system perspective of healthcare organizations.*

Furthermore, physicians are no exception to generational differences (Bujak).

Traditionalists and Baby Boomers

Traditionalists were born before 1945, and Baby Boomers were born between 1946 and 1964. These physicians look at medicine as a vocation, and their primary motivation for becoming physicians was respect for the unique role of healer. Traditionalists are trusting, hopeful, respectful, and loyal. Boomers tend to pursue status and tangible rewards more often, and are challenging, assertive, demanding, and more critical.

Generation X

Distinctly different from Traditionalists and Boomers, Generation X values a balanced lifestyle. Job security is important and loyalty is not valued, but they are concerned with frequency of call, work volume, salary, and perks. This generation is very techno-savvy and tend to work independently and delegate responsibility. They want to enhance their value in the marketplace (Bujak).

"It is impossible to hate someone whose story you know."

The physician's point of view

Every year, he worked harder and put in more hours, shuffling through the halls of the hospital as if dragging a ball and chain. He was a prisoner of his profession.

Tom was a physician who worked for a large HMO, which required his patients to leave the hospital within three days. This requirement created a lot of friction between Tom and the nurses. Every week it was something else—last week, physical therapy had scrawled in the progress note, "Pt. unsafe to go home." It ticked him off. As if his 10 years of medical school training didn't exist. As if any of his patients had ever fallen when they went home! Their blatant disregard for his training and judgment made the days heavier.

Recently, the nurses called his assistant to ask the same question they had asked Tom only 10 minutes before. They didn't realize that his and the assistant's desks faced each other, and that every time the nurses called, Tom's assistant would turn the phone around so that Tom could hear the same request all over again.

He thought of his uncle, who was a carpenter, and of how happy he was building cabinets his whole life. But as a carpenter of the human body, banging new knees and hips into place, Tom was harassed constantly by his boss, the nurses, and even the patients. His mind wandered to the scene yesterday with Mrs. Wright. On the first postop day, she was in pain and began to yell that she was going to sue him. Sue him? He was absolutely dumbfounded. Because she could not afford to pay, Tom had volunteered to do Mrs. Wright's hip surgery for free.

Needless to say, this was not the role he had imagined. This was not the way it used to be. He was tired of defending every little decision that came out of his mouth and tired of the constant battle.

When poor nurse-physician relationships characterize the work environment, the physician also loses. Not one person involved in the above situation felt good about his or her part in the drama. When such an atmosphere of frustration takes hold, creativity is stifled. The opportunity to have sustaining partnerships and meaningful relationships disappears. A physician loses something as basic as walking onto a floor and feeling respected and valued for what he brings to the team.

The same forces that have kept nurses subordinate for years create pressure for physicians to maintain their dominant position.

Female physicians

Remember your middle school playground? A group of boys in one corner and cliques of girls huddled in another, whispering their respective secrets. These groups of kids were established by varying degrees of "coolness," which were determined by unwritten rules known by all. Now, remember the kids who were always trying to fit in? That's how female physicians often feel.

Because female physicians are not the majority, they often feel as if they do not fit in. Males/physicians are the dominant group; females/nurses are the subordinate group. A female physician does not belong to either.

Female physicians are marginalized, and like any group of marginalized people, they are constantly trying to define their place—wherever that may be. Interestingly, yet not surprisingly, the first behavior any marginalized group will adopt is that of the dominant group. For this reason, we see female physicians who are gruff, bossy, demanding, etc., even though such a demeanor is stereotypically uncharacteristic of females. Acting this way typically produces an internal conflict for most female physicians. One female physician with whom I spoke had this to say about it all:

> *[Male physicians] want to be your best buddy, but can't stand that you are in "the club"—It's supposed to be a boys' club. If I give an order, I'm mean. If a male physician says the same exact words, he's taking charge of the situation like a real doctor.*

> *I was rounding with three other doctors in a neurosurgery rotation, and we were just about to leave the room when the patient looked at me and said, "Honey, can you get me some water?" Patients just assume I am the nurse.*

Because 50% of medical students are now women, this trend is changing. Nurses are frequently reporting that they enjoy collegial relationships with their female physician partners. But informal surveys show that only 15% of female physicians plan on working full time. This fact alone is projected to create a primary care physician shortage as female physicians seek positions in areas that do not have on-call demands, such as radiology, dermatology, and ophthalmology, in order to also raise families. In addition, waiting for a gender shift is not an option as all poor relationships affect patient safety today.

However, if a female physician does lash out at a nurse, we feel doubly betrayed because she is supposed to be "one of us." There is a part of us that simply can't believe one of our own can treat us that way. We do not innately recognize demanding, yelling and asserting to be female behaviors. But sometimes female doctors adopt these behaviors in an effort to fit in with male physicians.

Nurses

The agony

It is difficult to look at our wounds, acknowledge how despair has crept into our hearts in the workplace, and admit our disappointment with our profession and with ourselves. Every time we are part of a disruptive nurse-physician scene, we feel powerless because it is not possible to both remain quiet and be true to ourselves. We are robbed of our integrity and left in a state of moral anguish.

The deep wounds we feel are reflected in the current nursing shortage, which is actually a misnomer because it implies there are not enough nurses. It does not reflect the truth that nurses are actively leaving the profession. Imagine seeing the headline "NURSING EXODUS!" plastered across the front page of *The New York Times*. Such an impact would be far more profound—and accurate.

Nurses are leaving because their work environment is toxic. The work is physically, emotionally, and psychologically exhausting, and is so intense that there is often no time for the meals and breaks that nourish us. In fact, sustaining our energy in this environment is a constant challenge, especially because as human beings we also receive energy from good relationships, and nurses often lack those in the workplace. When they do exist, collegial and friendly relationships create an environment in which we can endure our difficult work. In a recent Clinical Advisory Board study of five destination hospitals, good relationships with coworkers was the number one reason that nurses gave for staying at a hospital.

Verbally abusive physicians add more poison to an already unhealthy scene. But it's not just the abusive and disruptive relationships that hurt us; it's the passive-aggressive doctor who consistently uses blue ink despite repeated reminders about the black-ink-only hospital policy. It's the doctor who totally ignores the dangerous abbreviations list.

Janice had floated to the medical floor where one of her patients was on isolation precautions. As she was walking down the hall, she saw the patient's physician writing orders while wearing an isolation gown. Concerned because the doctor typically wrote orders after leaving the room, Janice said, "Have you been in the room already?"

"Yes, I have," he replied brusquely.

"You are not supposed to come out of the isolation room in the gown," Janice said.

"I am well aware of that," he retorted, and kept writing. When finished with his charting, he walked back into the room and dropped the gown on the floor, signaling his blatant disregard for the rules and his contempt for the nurse who had the gall to question his actions.

Such events are painful. Every nurse of whom I ask a story takes but a second to recall a scene—even if it happened many years ago.

In crises, however—and such interactions are crises—there is also opportunity. For instance, when a close friend dies or a loved one receives the news that he or she has cancer, we are often inexplicably drawn to ask more spiritual or meaningful questions— the very nature of the event causes us to reach more deeply than usual (Watson, 2003). Likewise, painful nurse-physician interactions propel us to try to make sense of these hurtful relationships by starting with ourselves.

Powerlessness

Physicians are not the only ones causing disruptive relationships and producing an unfriendly environment—nurses are just more subtle in their aggression. If they have a problem, they tend not to address it directly. Nurses use a passive-aggressive communication style.

> *Recently, a nurse was scheduled for CPR training at 7:30 a.m., so that was exactly the time she arrived on the unit. When she arrived, the other nurses eyed the clock and shot furtive glances of disapproval in her direction for being late. Only then did she find out that, unbeknownst to her, she had been pulled from the class at the last minute and scheduled on the floor because a nurse had called in sick.*

These are good nurses—they are not aware of the damage they are causing. But this example illustrates how we lash out at each other and interact with physicians without first working out our own interaction skills. Many nurses do not realize that what makes them lash out is their own feeling of powerlessness.

Whenever there is a hierarchy and the group you belong to is not at the top of it, feelings of inferiority take hold. The energy that would normally be used to solve a problem is thwarted by these feelings, leaving the oppressed to take it out on each other openly or through passive aggression. Such responses occur when the charge nurse knows she needs another nurse to staff the floor safely, but no one listens, or when the staff nurse realizes that she cannot possibly cover another surgery. Their power and autonomy are stifled, so they direct their frustration toward each other.

As mentioned in Chapter 1, this kind of interaction is known as horizontal violence. "Horizontal violence drains nurses of vitality and undermines institutional attempts to create a satisfied nursing workforce" (Thomas, 2003). And it is these dynamics that keep nursing in the subordinate position—not physicians. It is our poor sense of self-esteem, individually and collectively, that prevents us from feeling empowered to change our situation (Roberts, 2000).

The way to improve nurse-physician relationships is to develop a high sense of self-esteem. To improve our collective self-esteem, each nurse must stand in awe of what she does, and she must recognize and value his/her tremendous work.

The ecstasy

Caring is at the heart of nursing. Watson (2003) says, "By attending to, honoring, entering into, and connecting with our deep humanity, we find the ethic and artistry of being, loving, caring" (2003). Recall an interaction with a patient that was particularly meaningful to you—the story you run home to tell your partner or pass along to your child or friend. This particular patient touched the very core of your being, and his or her story is etched in your heart. Take a moment to honor that connection.

Caring

> The call light was ringing before I was even out of report, so I decided to go directly to the patient's room. Anna was 40 years old and writhing in bed, both arms clenching her belly. "What's the matter?" I asked. "What can I do for you?"
>
> The patient glared and then responded sarcastically, "God help me! You don't know a damn thing, and you are supposed to be my nurse? Read the chart, girl! I have three ulcers. Can you read?" And then she proceeded to writhe and moan in agony.
>
> I walked over to the white board and picked up a blue marker. "What are their names?" I asked calmly. This just seemed to irritate her more.

                                       Speak Your Truth

> *"I don't know what you're talking about," she said.*
>
> *"Sure you do. Just give it a try," I replied. Her steel gaze pierced my back like a knife as I drew three different size circles on the board. Suddenly, she stopped moving. Arms still folded across her chest, she stared out the window, avoiding any eye contact to point out that she was still annoyed with me. But slowly her eyes jumped from the white board to the window and then back again to focus on the largest circle.*
>
> *"The biggest one," she said, "is my ex-husband, Bob." And so I wrote "Bob" in the circle. The smallest one was from the bills. I've since forgotten the other.*

With a little inspiration, I managed to help the two of us and helped her connect her life to her illness, making that very healing mind/body connection. From that moment on, Anna was "my" patient.

Something special happened in our story. It doesn't happen every day for a host of reasons—we are too busy, we have a patient who takes all of our energy, or the patient is completely unreceptive. Sometimes we are under too much stress and it is impossible to be present—not only for the patient, but for ourselves. But have you ever noticed that when we connect on a meaningful level with a patient, our own connection to all humanity seems heightened? Because fear, vulnerability, pain, and hopelessness are universal experiences, touching these emotions in a single person—to make just one patient feel better—feels like an act that serves the world.

Indeed, the very act of our caring, the art of connecting with another human being when he or she is in such a vulnerable position, is profoundly healing. But to connect fully with humanity in this way, we must first take a look at our own pain. We must call forth a deep and poignant scene with ourselves and acknowledge the damage that it and other poor nurse-physician relationships can cause.

Boundaries

We also must have a conversation with ourselves about the trouble we have maintaining boundaries. "Setting boundaries is an act of self love. At the center of sustaining our sense of purpose and personal power is our capacity to maintain boundaries. Boundaries give us a sense of empowerment" (Block, 2004). Caring for ourselves is necessary to our ability to heal because it takes a great deal of self-love to dissect such deep wounds and old scars.

Whenever we allow someone (e.g., a physician, spouse, or patient) to violate our personal boundaries, we lose power. It has never been a question of where to draw the line—everyone with whom I have spoken can state the exact moment when they felt small and insignificant. The question, rather, is what we do with the moment afterward. If we don't respond to this event, we are crippled.

To create healthy nurse-physician relationships, we must pay specific attention to the moment when physicians cross the line, and we must learn to respond in a different manner. Respecting and maintaining boundaries in this way is an act of self-love.

Adaptability

Over the past few years, the nurse's workload has steadily increased due to rising acuity and shortening lengths of stay, so our hospital adopted an acuity system that has greatly improved staffing. As I rounded the floor, several nurses seemed grateful, but there was something just below the surface that I couldn't put my finger on until we talked a bit more.

"It's just that ... well, I don't feel good," one nurse attempted to explain. After further probing, I discovered that some of the nurses felt guilty for having adequate staffing and being able to take meal breaks. I just had to tell them the story about the frogs.

If you put a frog into a pot of hot water, it will jump out immediately. But if you put a frog into a pot of cool water and then turn the heat up very, very slowly, it will boil to death. Like frogs, we humans are incredibly adaptable. And although adaptability has been a blessing over the years, it has been a curse as well, because when changes are slow and incremental, we don't really notice them and, without questioning them, automatically adapt. In this way, practices creep up on us. To what have we adapted over the years? These nurses had adapted to missed meals and breaks—so "cooler water" had become uncomfortable. How hot is the water in nursing?

A healing environment

As nurses, we not only care for patients but for our surroundings as well. We have a deep desire to make things better, which is one of the reasons we went into nursing. Healing is deeply embedded in the fabric of who we are. Nurses don't only heal patients, they attempt to heal the environment as well. But the negativity we absorb by continuously stressing over calming situations is not helpful to us, our profession, or our patients in the long run. The emotional and moral fatigue we suffer comes with too high a price.

> *Last week, Judy seriously questioned why she stayed in nursing at all—and she was not the only one. A pattern of ineffective communication had inconspicuously settled into the daily routine on the floor with one particular doctor. It was getting to the point where nurses would rather not care for his patients than deal with the confrontation that would surely ensue. Every interaction between this physician and the nurses ended in anger—sometimes tempers flared before they even saw each other.*

Mr. Smythe was four days postop after a hip surgery. He still felt nauseated and was refusing food. His bowel sounds were hypoactive, and he had a history of abdominal surgery and a previous ileus. Further, he kept ringing his call light asking the nurses to please help him. Despite the note on the front of the chart dictating these nursing concerns, Dr. Delaney made his rounds and wrote, "Discharge to home today," Mr. Smythe's nurse, Judy, felt totally ignored and, more important, she felt that the patient was in no shape to go home. After 20 years of experience, she thought at the very least an x-ray should be done. She had just explained this to Dr. Delaney when Megan, another nurse, rounded the corner and heard his response:

"I noticed something—the patient is OLD. Did you notice that? Did YOU go through 10 years of medical school? DID YOU? What makes you think for a minute that you know more than me?!" Judy turned and ran past Megan with a nosebleed. It was the worst abusive situation between a nurse and physician that Megan had ever seen—the blatant disregard for the nurse's assessment, the public critical attack, and the sarcasm were just too much. As soon as the doctor stormed off the floor, Megan opened the file cabinet and pulled out a quality variance sheet, intent on filling it out in detail. As she was writing, the social worker came up behind her and said, "Add my name to that; that was just horrible."

Nurse Managers

We need the help of caring nurses who are good at their jobs to heal nurse-physician relationships. Earlier, we remembered a special interaction with a patient and honored that moment as a universal portal that broadens our access to and appreciation for all humanity. We talked about the core of caring and the heart and soul of nursing—those moments that open the doors to a wider world. Nurse managers are in a pivotal position to help open that door to physicians.

The manager's experience

Dr. Delaney had only been in the manager's office for five minutes, and she could already tell that this conversation was going to be a challenge. His body language was too casual, as if he were sitting on a park bench in a photo shoot for Gentlemen's Quarterly *magazine.*

"I am following up on this problem," she said, showing him the quality variance report. "I understand that yesterday your interaction with Judy was so upsetting that she got a nosebleed. The problem is—"

"No," he interrupted, "the problem is that your nurses need tougher skins."

(This is usually the part where nursing leaves "the table." And why not? How do you find that shared pool of meaning after a remark like that? "Ten more minutes," she coached herself, and then looked into his eyes. "Never mind, five.") The conversation was still going nowhere, but he hadn't gotten up and left. Then she had an idea.

"I am sure you have heard Don Berwick say that 'every system is perfectly designed to get the outcome that it achieves'—it was first used by Toyota to describe the factories. What this means is that the factory is perfectly designed to produce the quality of car it produces. Well, your system of communicating with my nurses is perfectly designed to get the same results every single time you have a conversation—you will feel a lack of respect and trust, and they will feel ignored, hurt, and angry. Would you like to change the system?"

The room was still. Quietly, he said, "You don't think I see it in their eyes? You don't think I know that they think I am a lousy doctor?"

She told him the truth. "No, we didn't know you knew." Then, with more honesty than she could have hoped for, he shared his story. He explained that in the preop visit, the patient had already convinced himself that he was going to have an illness. He explained why he thought going home was the best option. He pointed out that there were 700 cc of urine in the Foley of a patient who had no IV and supposedly wasn't drinking.

"Could you communicate what you know and what you see with the nurses?" the manager asked. She then explained the nurses' concerns: The patient repeatedly asked for his doctor, saying he was in pain; the bowel sounded hypoactive; and he had a poor appetite.

When the doctor left her office more than a half-hour later, he was so quiet that the manager could not predict how this would turn out until the next interaction on the floor.

Anxiously, the staff had watched her door. After the doctor left, the manager took the time to talk to each of them individually about the incident and the doctor's explanation.

A few days later, Dr. Delaney was rounding with Megan. His first words were, "I understand that I need to communicate better."

"Yes, doctor," said Megan, "I think that's a good idea."

"You do understand that if I had been able to communicate, I wouldn't be divorced, don't you?" She smiled and said nothing. Together they assessed the patient.

As the physician turned to leave the floor, Megan called out "Doctor!" He turned around, and she continued, "We don't want to divorce you."

Conclusion

If only all problems with physicians could end in these crucial conversations. Then we would all value and respect each other more. In order to heal physician-nurse relationships, it is necessary to connect on this deep and meaningful level. By doing so, as when we connect with our patients, we connect with all humanity.

The first person we must connect with, however, is ourselves. Not until we admit our own pain and applaud the incredible work we do will we ever be able to change the pattern of harmful relationships. Ironically, it is in affirming "the agony and the ecstasy" of nursing that we will be able to change the current paradigm. When we realize the damage these disruptive relationships cause, we can protect ourselves better from them and react differently to them. When we realize the phenomenal work we do, we can break the cycle of oppression by raising our individual and collective self-esteem. In the end, the key stakeholders are all looking to be valued, to be respected, to belong, and to provide excellent patient care.

Perhaps it is only when we acknowledge how much pain and suffering there is in our broken hearts and broken spirits, our broken world—within and without—that we can return to that which is timeless that can comfort, sustain, and inspire/inspirit (Watson, 2003).

R E F L E C T I V E   E X E R C I S E

Acknowledgment

Identify one physician behavior that "shuts you down."

References

Block, P. (2004). "A Time to Heal." *Reflections on Nursing Leadership Quarterly* 4: 20–21.

Bujak, J. (2008). *Inside the Physician Mind: Finding Common Ground With Doctors*. Chicago: Health Administration Press, American College of Healthcare Executives.

The Joint Commission. (2010). "Sentinel Event Statistics." *www.jointcommission.org/ContinolEvents/Statistics* (accessed March 11, 2010).

Leonard, M., S. Graham, and D. Bonacum (2004). "The Human Factor: The Critical Importance of Effective Teamwork and Communication in Providing Safe Care." *Quality Safe Healthcare* 13 (Supp 1): 185–190.

Roberts, S. (2000). Development of a Positive Professional Identity: Liberating Oneself From the Oppressor Within." *Advances in Nursing Science* 22 (4): 71–82.

Thomas, S. (2003). Horizontal Hostility." *American Journal of Nursing* (103): 10.

Watson, J. (2003). Love and Caring: Ethics of Face and Hand—An Invitation to Return to the Heart and Soul of Nursing and Our Deep Humanity." *Nursing Administration Quarterly* 27 (3): 197–202.

Checking the Emotional Pulse
of Work Relationships

"No one can make you feel inferior without your consent."
—Eleanor Roosevelt

As with all nursing processes, we must begin by assessing the situation. So far, we have done so from a broad perspective by reviewing context, theory, and history. Now it is time to get down to business. It is time to narrow the focus from a collective to an individual standpoint—after all, poor nurse-physician relationships can only improve when you take ownership of and personal responsibility for your role in the problem.

The first step is to assess the quality of your work relationships. The second step is to assess barriers and individual responses to conflict. By taking the emotional pulse of the relationships on your unit, you will begin to understand why we respond the way we do to negative behavior. With this insight, you can learn to respond differently and change the existing culture.

Part I: Taking the Pulse of Nurse-Physician Relationships

Taking the pulse of physician relationships is a good starting point for change. Doing so allows you to dissect the current relationships in your facility and make sense of the problems you face.

In their research surrounding nurse-physician relationships, Marlene Kramer and Claudia Schmalenberg took a closer look at nurse-physician relationships by defining exactly what nurses meant when they described any nurse-physician relationship as "good." The term meant different things to different nurses, but the researchers did find that power consistently played a large role in the relationships (Kramer & Schmalenberg, 2003). They further developed the following five categories to define the types of relationship (Kramer & Schmalenberg, 2009):

1. Collegial—equal power, trust, and respect

2. Collaborative—mutual power, trust, and respect

3. Teacher-student—RN or MD can be either role; both willing to listen, teach, and learn

4. Friendly stranger—little trust and acknowledgement, courteous but formal

5. Hostile—adversarial and abusive; negativity in tone and action

Because the categories are based on a power difference, these scales tie in well with the oppression theory, which is also based on power.

Kramer and Schmalenberg also searched for a correlation between the quality of the physician-nurse relationships and the quality of patient care on a unit. They found that two out of the 14 ANCC Magnet Recognition Program® hospitals participating in the study had a formalized collaborative practice structure. Within these two hospitals, more than 75% of nurses rated their relationships as collegial. In other words, nurses rated the quality of care on the units with collaborative and collegial relationships significantly higher than they rated care on those units without such relationships.

A third observation was that relationships differ according to the service line. For instance, nurses in emergency and outpatient units reported more collegial relationships than those in the medical/surgical or critical care units (Kramer & Schmalenberg, 2003). In both the emergency and outpatient settings, the physician is more active on the unit and his presence more constant. Perhaps this increased amount of time together gives nurses and physicians an opportunity to break out of the MD-RN mold and relate on a more personal level.

It is important to acknowledge that collaboration is a relationship, a dynamic ongoing process. Yet when several studies were analyzed, collaboration was measured as an event (Schmalenberg et al, 2005). The AACN's "Standards for Establishing and Sustaining Healthy Work Environments" lays a solid foundation for practice and points out that collaboration must be viewed as a core value.

Collegial relationships

There are great doctors out there, and Jeff is one of them. He is a member of a special class of physicians that believes exchanging and sharing knowledge with one's colleagues (yes, that includes nurses) is an integral part of patient care. He treats all staff as if they are on the same team—and they are. He doesn't lash out at the nurses—not even after a patient has lashed out at him. He doesn't make nurses feel stupid when they call him in the middle of the night to inform him of a patient's changing status. His voice is steady, and he listens. Because of Jeff's congenial manner, nurses don't hesitate to ask questions; he makes them feel valued with his sincerity, and everything about him *invites* a conversation.

When writing orders, Jeff often explains his thought process so that those around him get the opportunity to learn. With this physician, nurses feel respected and acknowledged for their role as healthcare professionals—especially when he asks for their advice. When Jeff is around, the atmosphere is always comfortable.

Recently, for instance, Jeff had a difficult time determining whether a patient's pain medicine was working because he had just stepped onto the floor. But after checking the patient's pain flow sheet and speaking with the nurses, Jeff realized that his patient was always either awake and in pain or asleep. After sharing his findings with a nurse, she suggested switching the pain medicine in the patient-controlled analgesic from morphine to Dilaudid. After seeing improvement—a much more comfortable patient—due to the nurse's suggestion, Jeff exclaimed to the nurse, "Good call!"

In collegial relationships—such as those between Jeff and his nurse colleagues—the nurses and the doctor have mutual respect and power. Because of this, both parties feel empowered. When both nurses and physicians have power, they are better able to recognize the value in each other's education and experience. Doctors are respected for their years of training, and nurses are respected for their years of experience and for their assessment skills, derived from the vast amount of time they spend with patients.

For instance, the doctor acknowledges that during an eight- or 12-hour shift, a nurse can pick up on the subtle signs that lead to postop complications. Last week, one of Jeff's patients appeared to be suffering from the early signs of cardiac failure. A nurse picked up on the elderly patient's deteriorating condition and was able to act quickly, keeping the patient out of the ICU. Also, yesterday Jeff left in a hurry and forgot to write orders for a patient who was to have nothing by mouth in preparation for his surgery the next day. Jeff was grateful when the nurse caught the error in time so that the surgery could move forward as planned.

Within this environment, physicians and nurses consult each other frequently and seek each other's advice, to the full benefit of the patient. The nurses do not hesitate to ask questions or share opinions, and doctors listen and respond in a manner that encourages dialogue. Everyone must remember that knowledge is not solely the doctor's property. In fact, sharing knowledge openly allows for improved care, which is perhaps the most critical outcome of collegial relationships.

Brenda approached the doctor as he was leaving the floor. "Excuse me," she said, "but I think that continuing your patient's Toradol for four more doses might help her get a better handle on her pain—I noticed that her pain worsened after the order expired. Can we continue the Toradol?" It was a great idea, and even the physician agreed. In the end, it was the patient who benefited most.

The nurse manager also plays an important role in growing and promoting healthy nurse-physician relationships. Because of his or her supervisory role on the floor, the nurse manager is often responsible for setting the expectation for collegial relationships. He or she is in the perfect position to model the correct behavior and nurture relationships.

Collaborative relationships

Both collegial and collaborative relationships have their roots in the principles of collaboration, which is the art of working in partnership. The benefits of such relationships include positive patient health outcomes, decreased lengths of stay, and increased job satisfaction for both nurses and physicians. Collaboration begins with a vision shared by nurses, administration, and physicians and with clearly stated behavior expectations (LeTourneau, 2004).

> *Betina knew that her patient was reacting strongly to her medication, but she also knew that she had given her very little of it. When Dr. Renno arrived on the floor, he too was puzzled. Betina hesitated to offer her opinion because Dr. Renno had disagreed with an assessment she made last week. They brainstormed possible causes for the patient's heightened drug state. They discussed everything from increased creatine levels to drug sensitivity. Finally, Betina said, "I think this patient is taking her own pain medicine." Together, they went into the room and tried to help the groggy patient sit up in bed—and that's when the bottle of Percocet rolled to the floor.*

In a collaborative relationship, physicians and nurses participate together in the plan of care to produce positive outcomes for the patients. The nurses and physicians have a mutual respect for each other. The key difference between collegial and collaborative, however, is that the power is not equal. The nurses realize that, despite their input, the physician will always have the final say. For the most part, however, the power difference does not interfere with the working relationship, and both parties are able to work together for the benefit of the patient.

There is no debating the fact that collegial/collaborative relationships positively affect patient care. These relationships are not just about working together for the benefit of the patient; they are about a great relationship that is rewarding and energizing to both parties. People who have mutual trust and respect, as well as open communication, take their relationships beyond the work environment. They want to share a meal, have coffee, or celebrate milestones and holidays together. In Chapter 7, we will look at what structures and processes on an individual and organizational level create these relationships.

Teacher-student relationships

In teacher-student relationships, the physician or nurse takes on the role of mentor. Typically, the doctor educates the nurses. Often, however, the nurse is in a position to teach the physician what she has learned from her experience. Nurses generally have a wider, more holistic picture of patients and, historically, have been better able to consider the emotional and psychosocial aspects of patient care.

Although the nurse appreciates the information being shared—and although the outcomes are still beneficial for the patient—teacher-student relationships fall short of making both the nurse and the physician feel intrinsically good about their roles. Within these relationships, there is less trust, value, and respect than in collaborative and collegial relationships. This is because even though the teacher-student relationship may start off as a positive interaction between physicians and nurses, allowing the nurse to learn from the physician's years of schooling and helping the physician to better understand nursing's role in patient care, the relationship eventually takes its toll on the less powerful person involved, and negative feelings develop. The atmosphere may appear courteous and friendly, but both teacher and student lack authentic appreciation and respect for each other.

Kathy listened closely as Ms. Bryan complained. The patient was requesting a bolus of pain medication, but she had already taken 38 mg of morphine in the past six hours, so she was hesitant to give any more. Kathy did her assessment. Twelve hours postop after an anterior cervical operation, the patient could still not swallow water. "And I am upset with the doctor," the patient continued. "He just walked in the room, said, 'Guess you can't go home today,' and walked out. He didn't even look at my dressing!"

Sure enough, there were no orders written, so Kathy developed a plan of care. If she could get the patient to swallow, then she could start the longer-acting pain pills and get her patient's pain under control. So she called the doctor with a plan, unsure of how he would respond. "Can we get this patient on four doses of 10 mg of decadron IV to reduce the throat swelling and get her eating?" she asked. "Then I can get her pain under control with some longer-acting pills." He approved of the plan.

By the next morning, the patient had improved dramatically. The doctor stopped Kathy in the hall and asked, "Where did you learn that trick?"

"From the neurology doctors," she replied. "It works great." Thoughtfully, he nodded and left the floor.

Friendly stranger relationships

As Dr. Hughes walked by the nursing station, I watched all the nurses' facial expressions suddenly change to subtle smirks. I had seen this particular physician in action before, and I knew there was no threat of a flare-up or any other problematic confrontation—he never spoke to the nurses. Dr. Hughes simply came onto the unit, wrote orders, and left without speaking to anyone.

Relationships that used to require some form of intervention (e.g., used to be more teacher-student) have been replaced with more neutral relationships—or those that call for little interaction. Friendly stranger relationships evoke indifference. Such relationships originally cropped up in healthcare when, in an effort to increase productivity, hospitals decided to move the patient charts from the main nursing station to outside patients' rooms. Once that move occurred, the decline in communication between nurses and physicians was rapid and obvious.

Nurses and doctors used to congregate at the main hub and discuss potential problems. It was during these daily discussions that nurses could ask the doctors questions about their patients' plans of care, which fostered a learning environment. Now, however, a doctor can come to the floor, write orders, put up the yellow flag on the chart rack, and never speak to anyone. In that small effort to improve productivity, a daily opportunity to communicate was lost.

Linda was hoping to catch Dr. Horn before he left the floor, so she hovered outside of her patient's room where he was and caught up on her charting. Her patient was anxious because she had not received her necessary asthma inhalers or medications after surgery. When the doctor finished rounding with the patient, Linda said, "I noticed that none of the medications this patient was on prior to surgery have been restarted." For a moment, he glanced in her direction, and then resumed his charting. Linda wasn't sure what he would do, but much to her relief, she discovered after he left the floor that he had reordered the patient's meds.

Hostile relationships

Nurses report that negative patient outcomes occur more frequently when nurses interact with a difficult physician. Most of the scenarios in this book demonstrate negative interactions—and, unfortunately, they are all real-life examples. This is unfortunate as only 3%–5% of physician-nurse relationships are hostile, and these difficult relationships exponentially impact daily interactions on the unit.

After a doctor establishes a negative reputation for himself, nurses will go out of their way to avoid him. After all, no one wants to feel small, insignificant, or worthless. But the critical common thread in every disturbing physician-nurse interaction is that the patient loses.

Donna began nursing on the surgical floor only two years ago. She was just out of nursing school and still feeling her way around. When the manager asked for volunteers for the hospital's skin committee, she eagerly volunteered and enjoyed her role as a unit resource. The manager would call on her at staff meetings to share new information and report on hospitalwide efforts to decrease pressure ulcers.

One day while she was caring for a patient, Dr. Knowlten asked her to help with the wound care. Donna held the patient's leg while the doctor poured half a bottle of peroxide directly into the wound, causing the patient a great deal of pain.

After leaving the room, Donna asked to speak to the doctor. She told him about recent studies that showed hydrogen peroxide inhibited healthy cell development and about the latest recommendations. He replied, "Show me the data."

Donna was excited. Here was her chance to contribute to a practice change that would benefit all of Dr. Knowlten's patients. She spent more than two hours pulling up research and gathering all the pertinent information.

The next day, she proudly handed her work to Dr. Knowlten. But he didn't even look at it. He plopped the papers on the counter and said, "Donna, can you help me?" Then he walked into the same patient's room and proceeded to pour an entire bottle of peroxide into the wound.

For the next four years, Donna never made another suggestion to Dr. Knowlten. Finally, on the day she quit, she told her manager about the situation and about the fact that every time she saw that doctor, she just turned her head and looked the other way. She shared how painful it was to even look at him because it reminded her of that day, when she had truly gotten her hopes up. She had thought that she had an opportunity to improve patient care and was unprepared for the doctor's arrogant and humiliating response. Donna felt like she had been set up, and the feeling of betrayal was not easily forgotten.

Such stories share a common denominator: the hostile physician. For this particular doctor, internal and external factors were at play when he became agitated. Sometimes the way a nurse presented a suggestion would set him off, or the weight of his personal problems would cause him to erupt. Either way, this once disruptive physician now has better relationships with the nurses—some more than others, of course. Some speculate that his softening came with age—perhaps time has given him a greater understanding of the nurse's role and a greater appreciation for her work. But let's not forget that with age comes experience, and some experiences serve as the ultimate eye-openers.

The nurses were at the main station when Dr. Knowlten arrived on the floor. He asked gruffly, "Have you gotten my patient out of bed yet?" It was 10:00 a.m.

"No," the nurse responded. "Your patient is very heavy, and I thought it better to wait for physical therapy to help in a half hour."

"Nonsense. You girls are just lazy," he said as he stomped off to see his patient.

Several minutes later, the doctor yelled frantically from the patient's room, "Help! Help!" They all rushed into the room to find Dr. Knowlten pinned to the bed under his heavy patient.

Relationship Tips

If the relationship is collegial:

- Personally thank the physician publicly

- Send a thank-you note to him/her

- Copy the medical director and CEO

- **Tip:** Be specific; give examples of collaboration that improved patient outcomes

© 2010 HCPro, Inc.

If the relationship is collaborative:

- The goal is to increase trust and respect. This takes time.

- "Show your stuff." For example:

  - Use progress notes to indicate that you are aware of the physician's main concern about the patient, as well as your interventions

  - Ask questions and share concerns

  - Use every event as a learning opportunity and debrief cases often

If the relationship is teacher-student:

- The goal is to develop a relationship that doesn't exist solely around work

- Learn about each other as human beings: Explore topics such as hobbies or vacations

- Plan joint educational and celebratory events

If the relationship is friendly stranger:

- Most difficult to reach, so start with daily contact: eye contact, names first

- Don't play the game; engage in conversation

- Look for common educational opportunities (e.g., ask to be mentored in a specific area or procedure)

If the relationship is hostile:

- Never tolerate the behavior

- Always say, "May I speak to you for a moment in private?"

- Explain the physician behavior and state its effect

- Always first take your issues directly to the physician

- If that doesn't work, report to manager and copy the medical director

Part II: Taking the Pulse of the Physicians

Physicians know their own behavior. They could categorize themselves and their peers in a heartbeat. I was joking with a physician with whom I work very closely when he asked for a copy of this book. "Do you want the copy with all of the real names in the margin?" I asked.

"No, I'm certain I can tell who they are," he replied. "In fact, why don't you read several of these vignettes out loud at weekly rounds, and we can all shout out the names!"

Several months ago, I visited a hospital and talked to the nurses on a pediatric intensive care unit. I had heard from other staff that there was a disruptive doctor who had been harassing nurses for more than fifteen years. When I brought the subject up, one nurse reluctantly began telling her story:

> *"I get a visceral feeling in my gut whenever I see him," she started slowly while holding her stomach. "Last week he came onto the unit and took one look at my haircut and said something horrible. I told him not to speak to me that way, and he responded by cursing at me and walking off the floor. We don't bother reporting it anymore after years of reporting it and having nothing happen."*

They "know," but they don't do anything. Many medical directors feel strongly that to report their peers' transgressions is an act of betrayal. Why? Because deeply engrained in the physician culture is a sacred pact to keep each other safe. In our sue-happy society, we don't make being a doctor easy, and we don't nurture a culture where it's okay to talk about your mistakes. So when staff nurses and managers report issues to the medical director and nothing happens, they are perplexed. And because nothing happens, the behavior continues because the medical directors feel impotent and nursing feels hopeless.

> *The room was filled with emergency room physicians, and so I took the opportunity to ask a question. "Why didn't any of you speak up when you saw Bill yelling at the triage nurse or when you saw John dragging his feet on a patient who should have been expedited to the cath lab?" The room was very quiet. Finally a physician said, "Because someday, that irate doc could be me. And since I need my peers to cover my back, I'm going to cover theirs."*

Relationships are complex and dynamic. Although we cannot control physicians' perceptions, their personal problems, or our history, we always have control over how we respond to them. Nurses who will not tolerate disruptive behavior are the "Aunt Janes." According to S. J. Roberts' article, "Development of a Positive Professional Identity: Liberating Oneself From the Oppressor Within," Aunt Janes are nurses who articulate a shared vision of providing excellent care and insist on collegial relationships. In short, they "speak their truth" no matter what. They have found their power and are helping change the culture. Aunt Janes are discussed in depth in Chapter 6.

Take a minute to think about the physicians with whom you work, or the physicians with whom you wish you had a better relationship. As in the story above, one physician's behavior can fit into more than one category, and all nurse-physician relationships fit into at least one particular category. Because each is its own combination, remember that the best way to improve nurse-physician relationships is one relationship at a time. Use Figure 1 as a pulse-taking exercise.

FIGURE
1
Pulse-Taking Exercise

In the blanks below, write the names of the five doctors with whom you interact most frequently or who raise the hairs on your neck:

1. _____

2. _____

3. _____

4. _____

5. _____

Now list the above names in the appropriate box:

Collegial

Collaborative

Teacher-student

Pulse-Taking Exercise (cont.)

Friendly stranger

Hostile

And remember ...
Collegial: Equal-power relationships
Collaborative: Good working relationship, but the doctor has more power
Teacher-student: Centers around communication of knowledge
Friendly stranger: Near absence of any relationship
Hostile: Interactions leave you feeling worthless; negative patient outcomes

Possible follow-up actions to above
After reviewing what you've written in the boxes above, make an action plan for improving those relationships. Start by implementing some of the following suggestions:

If collegial, send an e-mail or thank-you note saying how much you enjoy your working relationship. Nominate the physician for an award.

If collaborative, provide opportunities for brief unit inservices to discuss particular cases and increase knowledge base. Advocate for joint education. Attend rounds daily. Perform a review of a difficult case and invite physicians and nurses to it. Form multidisciplinary teams to create standards. Also, send thank-you notes and plan social events to increase opportunities for communication.

If teacher-student, encourage physician-nurse inservices. Include your recommendation for treatment in the conversations. State that you would like to have a more collaborative relationship and that you believe this will help all involved—the patient, the nurse, and the physician. To develop trust and respect, round with the physician and see how your assessment and plan of care compare to that of the physician. Create opportunities for collaboration and socialization.

 Speak Your Truth

FIGURE 1

Pulse-Taking Exercise (cont.)

If friendly stranger, you must first establish a relationship. Do so by using humor, social events, or conversation to bring the physician out of his shell. Encourage conversation and find a common connection. Ask the manager to intervene and have one-on-one dialogue with the physician. Publicly state shared vision of collaboration at physician meetings. Take friendly stranger interactions into collaborative interactions.

If hostile, take a firm stance on disruptive physician behavior by insisting on a zero-tolerance policy. Hospital or clinic administrators must state behavioral expectations clearly. Create solidarity on the unit. Nursing management, administrators, and physician champions must form a strong alliance. Always try to resolve the situation yourself first. If you are unable to resolve issues on the unit, "write up" unacceptable behavior and copy to peer review. Speak your truth.

Part III: Taking Your Own Pulse

We must acknowledge our own behavioral patterns.

I have known Mary for eight years. We were roommates on a traveling nurse assignment in Southern California and became fast friends. Mary is a neonatal intensive care nurse (and now mother), and in all our conversations over the years, she never once mentioned a problem with physician relationships—until now.

"Are there any problems with physician and nurse relationships on your unit?" I asked curiously.

"Why, yes, all the time," she responded, matter of factly.

"Why didn't you mention this to me before?"

"Because I just ignore them," she admitted. "I just focus all my energy on my baby ... and I tune them out."

We talked for a long time. The thought had never occurred to Mary that the healthy, healing environment she wanted for the infants on her unit was directly affected by these poor relationships—that just focusing on her baby was not the optimal situation for patient safety or for her own personal satisfaction. "I never thought about it that way," she reflected. Everyone she worked with responded to disruptive behavior the same way she did—by ignoring it and hoping it would go away.

As she told me stories of "men behaving badly," I encouraged her to address their poor behavior. "You want me to do what?" she exclaimed. "No way!"

No way

Most nurses do not like conflict; few feel prepared to deal with confrontation, and many handle the problem by avoiding it. For nursing to survive, however, nurses must learn how to deal constructively with conflict. In her article "Professional Development: 'Horizontal Hostility,' " Thomas says, "Research shows that nurses who report the greatest degree of conflict with other nurses also report the highest rates of burnout" (2003).

Remember how terrifying it was to trust that the water would hold you up when you learned how to swim? Or how anxious you were during those first few weeks of driving? As with any skill, engaging in constructive confrontation becomes easier with practice, and the first time is always the most difficult. Conquering your fear of confrontation is necessary because no one is going to solve your poor nurse-physician relationship problems for you. **The person who will change the culture is you.**

It is our moral and ethical responsibility to take the first step toward change individually so that we can shift the paradigm collectively. We must identify the forces that make us exclaim apprehensively, "No way!"

Fear and uncertainty

Courage is integrity put forth to the world. The root word for courage is "Coeur," from Latin, meaning "from the heart." It takes courage to stand up for yourself to someone you perceive as more powerful than you. It takes courage to speak to someone who has consistently silenced you in the past. When we speak from our heart, we are speaking our truth. Veracity takes hold, and we are empowered.

There is always tremendous risk in acting differently because we could be wrong, ridiculed, or worse, ignored. We feel vulnerable because we can't predict the outcome. But this is human nature. To change the pattern of abusive physician-nurse relationships, we need moral courage.

I recently spoke during a conference about building community within a hospital and was disappointed at the questions asked afterward. The audience wanted to know the exact recipe for making a community, rather than wanting to really understand the need for belonging—as if performing a set of actions scribbled on a notepad would guarantee community. The truth is that there is no quick fix to creating a better community, a sense of belonging and pride, or healthy nurse-physician relationships. Courage and creativity are required to shift these relationships which are deeply embedded in culture. Overcoming cultural and power differences requires that your heart be present and that you actively care. The secret to change is having a raised awareness of the current situation in your organization and in your life, and having the self-love and courage to maintain healthy boundaries.

Any activity that increases communication, education, and socialization among nurses and physicians, with the common vision of great patient care, is a winner. There are plenty of Aunt Janes out there right now, and none of their strategies were from a recipe card—they simply spoke their truth from their hearts.

Judy was the only night nurse in a busy emergency room. She had been on the job for only a few months, and she was already tired of one particular physician's irate and degrading behavior. One night, he said something that pushed her so far that she can't even recall the comment now. She was so enraged that she swept the charts off the counter and within seconds she was laying supine on the counter, holding a potted plant against her belly as though the doctor's actions had put her six feet under. The following scene unraveled:

Doctor: *What the hell do you think you're doing? Knock it off!*

Nurse: *I am mortally wounded.*

Doctor: *Knock it off and get to work!*

Nurse: *No, not until you say you are sorry.*

Doctor: *Okay. I'm sorry.*

Nurse: *No, you have to mean it.*

Doctor: *Oh, knock this OFF! ....Okay, I'm sorry.*

Judy got down from the counter. Following this incident, the two continued to work together for years. To this day, she claims that he taught her more than anyone else and that he alone is responsible for making her a terrific nurse—which could only occur after Judy's antics smoothed out their rocky beginning and she successfully drew the line. We can learn a tremendous amount from physicians, but only when we have a relationship with them.

Maintaining our boundaries

The line is the boundary that physicians cross over when they treat you as less than the professional, competent, caring nurse you are. As mentioned before, maintaining your boundaries is an act of self-love. The bottom line is that you must care enough for yourself—you must have enough compassion for yourself—that you simply cannot stay in an abusive situation.

Sometimes caring for yourself is a much greater challenge than caring for others. Every time physicians cross the line, there is a conflict. Each one of these times, you make a choice: tell no one and internalize the conflict, or speak your truth and allow for discussion and closure. How you decide to respond determines the quality of relationships you will have with our physician partners.

Unfortunately, avoidance is the most popular style of dealing with conflict for both nurses and physicians. In the "Silence Kills" studies, 84% of physicians saw a coworker taking shortcuts that could be dangerous to a patient, yet less than 10% confronted colleagues. Another researcher coined the phrase "self silencing" while studying confrontation for women. She found that women value their relationship with each other more than anything else and to keep the peace, they keep quiet (Jack, 1991). People respond differently to conflict because we do not all value the same things. Some people believe in keeping the peace at any cost, while others place more value on the task at hand. Still others believe that the goal is paramount and will forsake the relationship to reach their goal.

The Bartol/McSweeney conflict management scale is based on J. Hall's conceptualization of conflict (Hall, 1973). Rather than resolving or eradicating conflict, these authors see conflict as a potential source of growth if nurses recognize their own style and use it to promote positive change (Bartol, 2001).

Think of the last confrontation you had with a physician. Review the following ways people deal with conflict and circle the one you most commonly use. Most people will try one way first and, if it does not work, will resort to another (Parrish & Bartol, 1998). Which is your primary conflict style, and which is your default?

Collaborative: You value the relationship and the goal to be accomplished

Compromise: You believe you must give a little to get a little

Accommodation: You believe you should relinquish your goals to maintain a relationship

Forcing: You value the task at hand or goal as most important

Avoidance: You believe that efforts to resolve conflict are useless; neither the goal nor the relationship is worth the conflict

What would Jane do?

Jane sees a problem.

Jane tells Dick.

Dick is mean—Dick crosses over the boundary line! What's your conflict style?

Jane goes silent (avoidance).

Jane stays quiet because it will interfere (compromise).

Jane refers to hospital policy (forcing).

Jane states how she feels and proceeds (collaborative).

Jane does what the physician says (accommodation).

A Story of Courage and Confrontation

Sally dreaded calling the physician. At morning rounds, he had told her that he wrote prescriptions and put them in the chart. She had searched everywhere and had scrutinized the chart before calling his office again. When she told him that she could not find the prescriptions, he began yelling, "I told you where they were; it's your problem, and I am not writing out more prescriptions for you." He hung up.

Sally asked the charge nurse to help her search the patient's room and the floor and to double check that the prescriptions were not in the chart. She could not discharge the patient without the pain medication. When she called back, he yelled again, "I am not writing them out for you again!" This time, however, he had crossed the line.

Sally interrupted him. "Please stop saying that. The prescriptions are not for me, they are for OUR patient, whom I am trying to help. This has nothing to do with me. I am simply trying to get our patient's pain medication so he can go home."

What will Jane do?

Here is Jane's shining moment. Physician-nurse relationships will improve only to the extent that nurses change their current response. Jane must break the pattern in order for the culture of domineering physicians to become extinct. Once aware of her pattern of dealing with conflict, Jane dares to try a different method—all patterns of behavior can be broken by the understanding that there is another pattern available.

For example, let's say that you travel the same route to work every day. One day, some-one tips you off about a shortcut. You decide to change your route, or pattern, and take the shorter, better route and experience positive results. Understanding that disruptive nurse-physician relationships are harmful to both patients and nurses—and recognizing the dominant and oppressive forces that have been shaped by centuries of behavior—raises our awareness and opens us up to taking the better route, or changing our pat-terned responses.

Jane has a lot of options:

- Jane just can't keep quiet

- Jane writes up an incident report

- Jane state the behavior is unacceptable

- Jane consults her managers

- Jane tells Dick to stop

- Jane reminds Dick of the new behavioral standards

- Jane tells Dick that his comment was rude and that his caustic remarks make it difficult to have a collegial and professional relationship

Figure 2 contains an exercise that will help you prepare for conflict.

Splash! Exercise

There is no optimal way to deal with conflict. Just like heading into a pool of cold water, it doesn't matter if you jump in or climb slowly down the ladder—you've got to go for it. The critical part is that you get into the water. The following exercise will be more meaningful if you remember an actual event from the past. Jump in and play along:

1. Use the blank spaces in this tool to jot down the names of the physicians who are in the Neutral or Negative categories from the exercise you did in Figure 1.

2. In the space for this, write down how you feel when in this physician's presence.

3. Next, list the specific behavior that intimidates you or examples of when this physician has crossed over the line.

4. Write down your conflict style.

5. If you continue in the same pattern, the relationships on your unit will also follow that pattern. Can you think of new responses or creative options?

Review the following example of the Splash! exercise before beginning:

Physician:	Dr. Rude
Feeling:	Hurt/angry
Physician behavior:	Obnoxious and loud
My conflict style:	Avoidance
My typical response:	Leave—ASAP!
New response:	Ask to speak to him alone, or ask my manager
	to come with me

FIGURE
2

Splash! Exercise (cont.)

Physician:

Feeling:

Physician behavior:

My conflict style:

My typical response:

New response:

Physician:

Feeling:

Physician behavior:

My conflict style:

My typical response:

New response:

Physician:

Feeling:

Physician behavior:

My conflict style:

My typical response:

New response:

References

Bartol, G.M., et al. (2001). "Effective Conflict Management Begins With Knowing Your Style." *Journal for Nurses in Staff Development* 17 (1): 34–40.

Hall, J. (1973). *Conflict Management Survey.* Conroe, TX: Teleometrics Int'l.

Jack, D. (1991). *Silencing the Self: Women and Depression.* New York; Harper.

Kramer, M., and C. Schmalenber (2003). "Securing 'Good' Nurse Physician Relationships." *Nursing Management* (7): 34–38.

Larson, E. (1999). "The Impact of Physician-Nurse Interactions on Patient Care." *Holistic Nursing Practice* 3 (2): 38–46.

LeTourneau, B. (2004). "Physicians and Nurses: Friends or Foes?" *Journal of Healthcare Management* 49 (1): 12–16.

Parrish, R., and G. Bartol (1998). *The Relationship of Conflict Management Styles to Selected Personality Characteristics.* Paper presented at the meeting of the 10th International Nursing Research Congress, Utrecht, The Netherlands.

Roberts, S. J. (2000). "Development of a Positive Professional Identity: Liberating Oneself From the Oppressor Within." *Advances in Nursing Science* 22 (4): 71–82.

Schmalenberg, C., and M. Kramer. (2009). "Nurse-Physician Relationships in Hospitals: 20,000 Nurses Tell Their Story." *Critical Care Nurse* 29 (1).

Schmalenberg, C., et al. (2005). "Excellence Through Evidence: Securing Collegial/Collaborative Nurse-Physician Relationships, Part I." *Journal of Nursing Administration* 35 (10): 450–458.

Thomas, S. (2003). "Professional Development: 'Horizontal Hostility.' " *Advanced Journal of Nursing* 103 (10): 87–91.

Vitalsmarts. (2005). "Why Silence Kills." *www.silencekills.com* (accessed March 15, 2010).

Breakdowns and Opportunities

LEARNING OBJECTIVES

After reading this chapter, the participant will be able to:

- List key steps used for calling difficult physicians on the telephone

- Explain how administrative support, a zero-tolerance policy, and assertiveness training are used as opportunities for improving nurse-physician relationships

- List and describe two practical strategies for nurturing relationships on your unit

"We have an obligation to work together to define the next level of relationship."
—*Lazar J. Greenfield, MD (1999)*

Every breakdown in communication is an opportunity for growth. Communication breakdowns occur all the time because physicians and nurses see the world from different perspectives. Physicians, for example, consistently report a higher degree of collaboration with nurses than nurses report. A literature review of physician-nurse issues from 1990–1995 found that 64% of the citations were reported in nursing journals and only 29.5% were found in medical journals.

Physicians and nurses also have varying perspectives about the very components of collaboration and communication (Larson, 1999). Doctors rated their attitudes and behaviors toward nurses more highly than the nurses rated them, and when confronted, several physicians appeared genuinely surprised to learn that the nurses found their behavior unacceptable (Copnell, 2003). Even though a high percentage of both physicians and nurses believed that collaboration was important, only 27% of those same nurses reported they actually had collaboration (Ferrand, 2003). Clearly, there is a huge gap to traverse before we can improve our relationships. Even cultural differences between physicians and nurses were found to be significant in incident reporting. Nurses reported more frequently because the nursing culture provides directives to do so, while physicians preferred keeping incidents "in house" (Kingston, 2004).

> *"Here's my problem," said the unit manager. "When I survey the physicians, they say that relationships with the nurses are 'great.' Then I survey the nurses and they say the same thing—only I don't believe them, because I can see on a daily basis that MD-RN relationships on my unit have a long way to go. But where do I start when both groups act satisfied with the status quo?"*

There is not even agreement about something as basic as the nurse's role. "There is a fundamental difference in the perception of what the role of nursing ought to be," says Greenfield in his article, "Doctors and Nurses: A Troubled Partnership" (1999). Our common experience tells us that our "appropriate functions" vary according to the time of day. If it's noon, the nurse had better not make a decision to increase or change medications or he or she will hear, "You're not the doctor." If it is midnight, the nurse had better make a decision or he or she will hear, "Why did you bother to call me? You know what to do."

We appear to disagree over roles, collaboration, attitudes, behavior, incident reporting, and styles of communication. With all of these documented differences, how do we move forward?

By focusing on our common ground: the patient. A shared vision of excellent quality care must be repeatedly articulated. Physicians and nurses must create this vision based on mutual values (Larson, 1999). For example, I recently worked on a project to standardize postoperative orders, and whenever there was significant disagreement, the conversation turned to best practice. Physicians and nurses could reach consensus more easily by asking the question, "What does the evidence and research say about best practice?"

When in conflict, disagreements become clearer when the focus is on what's best for the patient. Then it becomes not about our respective roles or actions but about what the patient needs. Therefore, in words and behavior, nurses and physicians must consistently remind each other of the common goal: to provide excellent, safe, quality care for the patient.

Breakdowns in Communication

Disagreements over discharge orders

When nurses and physicians don't communicate about the discharge plan, neither understands the other's concerns, and there is likely to be last-minute conflict. Once in such a conflict, the only way out is to communicate.

Samantha knocked on the manager's door. "He's done it again," she said. Sam was referring to one of the physicians—who once again was discharging to home a patient who couldn't even walk from the chair to the bathroom. To make matters worse, she said, "I asked him for a home health order, and he refused to give one. I'm getting tired of this."

The manager went to find the doctor, who was already irate because this situation had occurred before. "Do whatever you want," he said as the manager approached him.

"It's not about what I want or what the nurses want," she said. "It's about the patient."

From there, the conversation's focus shifted. The physician explained his concern that the patient would contract a healthcare-acquired infection at a skilled nursing facility and was too weak to handle another setback. The nurse manager explained Samantha's concern that, if the patient went home, she could fall as she tried to get to the bathroom.

Once each understood the other's perspective, the doctor ordered home health, and the patient's recovery was uneventful.

One way to avoid such discharge problems from the beginning is to have the physician communicate the plan for discharge at the time of admission or on the day of surgery. In our hospital, the standardized postoperative order forms have been changed so that the first line reads: "Anticipate discharge to _____. Estimated length of stay _____ days."

Having such a plan and working out the concerns in the early stages is a lot less stressful than trying to communicate a different plan with the physician just minutes before discharge. With this system, there is no guessing about what the physician wants; there is plenty of time to bring up concerns, and everyone is literally on the same page.

Disagreements over treatment decisions

How nurses and physicians communicate about treatment depends on the relationship. If it is collaborative, speaking up and sharing concerns is appreciated and is often an opportunity for both parties to learn something new. If it is neutral or negative, it is more difficult to make yourself heard. In either case, however, if you disagree with a treatment decision, base your actions on the safety of—or danger to—the patient.

If the patient's life is in danger, take action by following the chain of command: manager, chief of practice, medical director, etc. In general, there is more danger for the patient in keeping quiet than in sharing your concerns. If your concerns are not warranted, then at the very least you learn something—and the physician usually does, too.

Cary called the physician at 1 a.m. to inform him of the postop patient's incredibly high lab value. She couldn't believe that he didn't issue any stat orders. "Maybe he wasn't really awake," the day nurse commented, and then called him again at 7:30 a.m.

"I know," said the doctor. "They already called me at 1 a.m.!" He still did nothing.

At this point, the patient was in serious danger. The lab values indicated he would have a serious bleed out. Blood was already oozing from the IV line, and the IV nurse had been called to redress and sandbag the arm. The situation was critical, and the attending was not responsive.

Another physician was consulting on the case. The nurses had a great relationship with him, so they called him stat—and he responded stat. Within minutes, he was on the floor giving orders as staff ran to the blood bank for fresh frozen plasma and to the pharmacy for the much-needed Vitamin K.

Incidents of disruptive physician behavior

According to nurses, disruptive physician behavior most often occurs after they place phone calls to physicians, after they ask questions or seek clarification of physician orders, when physicians feel their orders were not carried out correctly or in a timely manner, when there are perceived delays in care, and when there are sudden changes in patient status (Rosenstein, 2002).

Physicians believe the primary cause of their disruptive behavior is when their orders are not being carried out correctly or in a timely manner (Rosenstein, 2002). Nurses depend on the actions of personnel in other departments; physicians often perceive a delay in medication administration or delivery of supplies as ineptitude on the part of the nurse. When studying the nurses' work, researchers found that nurses experience an average of 8.4 system interruptions per eight-hour shift (Tucker). Therefore, managers must follow up on delays or incorrect treatment. If they do not, physicians will be left to draw their own conclusions, which will most likely be that "it was the nurse's fault."

And there's always one thing in common with bad scenes: a tremendous amount of emotional charge. No one can solve a problem in the midst of so much hurt and anger.

The answer is to disengage—to physically remove yourself and others from the verbal abuse—and return to the issue at a later date.

Faye tried to hold on to the squirming baby. The physician's first two attempts at a lumbar puncture had already failed. And then he missed for a third time.

Faye put the baby back in its crib and took off her gloves. "What do you think you're doing?" yelled the doctor. "Get back here!"

"No," she replied. "That's enough."

"I will have you fired," he said, shaking his finger wildly. "I will report you to the CEO, and you will have to answer to him."

"Fine," said Faye as she left the room.

Two days later, Faye and the doctor sat in front of the CEO. The doctor ranted loudly, stating his case for several minutes. Then it was Faye's turn. She said only one sentence: "If that was your son, would you have wanted the nurse to hold him for yet a fourth try at a lumbar puncture?"

The doctor was caught off-guard. "No," he answered hesitantly. "If that were my son, I would have wanted you to do exactly what you did."

Like Faye, refuse to stand by and allow yourself to be affected by the abuse. Instead, try any of the following:

- Page the manager or medical director

- Call your hospital's code for disruptive behavior

- Take the conversation off the floor

- Refuse to participate if the physician is yelling

- Tell the physician you will make an appointment with him and his chief so that you can all discuss the issue later

A critical response to highly emotional situations is to disengage until emotions have calmed and all parties can be more objective.

Telephone trouble

Physicians often act like a nurse's phone call is a huge interruption—without realizing that the call interrupts the nurse's day as well. Keep the following telephone tips in mind:

- Don't begin with an apology. Identify yourself and the patient.

- Always have the chart, labs, and latest vital signs in hand.

- Put yourself in the physician's shoes; use critical thinking skills and have an idea of what you think is needed before you call.

- Consult other nurses if necessary, especially for after-hours calls and if you are a new nurse.

- Don't beat around the bush; say what you need or want.

- Anticipate after-hours needs as much as possible so you won't need to call a physician.

- Use read-backs—repeat back to the physician a summary of the order or the conversation.

- Use the speakerphone for rude physicians, and let them know you are doing so.

- If a physician is verbally abusive, say, "I am hanging up now. Please call back when you are calmer." Then hang up.

The SBAR tool for preventing breakdowns

According to Dr. M. Leonard, et al. (2004) communication breakdown between nurses and physicians often occurs when they do not have a set system or tool for communication. "All too frequently, effective communication is situation or personality dependent. Other high-reliability domains, such as commercial aviation, have shown that the adoption of standardized tools and behaviors is a very effective strategy in enhancing teamwork and reducing risk" (Leonard, Graham, & Bonacum, 2004).

After examining the different ways nurses and physicians communicate, Leonard's team developed a tool that would give each group exactly what it needed. The physicians received clear, concise information, and the nurses were empowered to state their needs and opinions. The tool is a predictable, formalized way of communicating that helps develop critical thinking skills and has been successfully applied in obstetrics, rapid-response teams, ambulatory care, intensive care, and other areas.

This tool, known as SBAR (Situation, Background, Assessment, Recommendation), streamlines the way in which nurses and physicians seek and share information during telephone calls. To use it, the nurse must answer the following questions before contacting the physician so that he or she is fully prepared to give answers and make recommendations about the patient's condition:

Situation: What is going on with the patient?

Background: What is the clinical background or context?

Assessment: What do I think the problem is?

Recommendation: What would I do to correct the problem?

The following is a clinical example from Leonard's (2004) article:

Situation: "Dr. Preston, I'm calling about Mr. Lakewood, who's having trouble breathing."

Background: "He's a 54-year-old man with chronic lung disease whose health has been sliding downhill, and this morning, he is acutely worse."

Assessment: "I don't hear any breath sounds in his right chest. I think he has a pneumo-thorax. Respirations 28."

Recommendation: "I need you to see him right now. I think he needs a chest tube."

One of the most exciting elements of this tool is that a nurse can ask a physician to come see the patient. To make this element even more useful, Leonard's team has made it standard safety practice in perinatal care for the physician to come into the hospital when the nurse is worried or concerned. "The situation is not open to argument at the time that the request is made, particularly at night or on weekends; if the relationship needs to be reassessed, that can be carried out sometime in the future when people can be more objective" (Leonard, 2004).

In this way, our feeling that something is wrong is validated without the physician pressuring us to convince him that the situation is serious. The old pattern of beating around the bush creates a great deal of stress and predisposes the patient to injury. In the worksheet they created to shed light on the issue, Knox and Simpson (2004) say, "In cases resulting in medical accident or patient injury, physicians are often quoted as saying, 'If she had only told me this was a real emergency, I would have come right in, but I didn't know things were that bad.' "

All nurses will tell you they had bad feelings about a patient before his or her health went downhill. Such intuition can be of vital importance and can, in fact, save lives. Speaking up is therefore critical to creating a safe environment, but it is only half the solution. What we say must also be heard. We must use the opportunities created by communication breakdowns to change the culture so that nurses will speak their truth and physicians will be receptive to it.

 Speak Your Truth

Conveying information and hearing that information is so important that when The Joint Commission analyzed sentinel events in a Midwestern hospital, it found that communication was a factor in 65% of sentinel events and 90% of root cause analyses. The hospital implemented a spread team of doctors and nurses to increase awareness and provide SBAR education. The results? A decrease in adverse events per 1,000 patient days from 89.9% to 29.9%. In addition, the hospital's use of SBAR exceeded 90% in the first year (Raica).

Opportunities for Improvement

Opportunities for improving communication between physicians and nurses pop up every day. You find them in the irate doctor who belittles a nurse right in front of her patient, or in the physician who refuses to call nurses by name. It is during these unfortunate events that the chance to speak your truth arises.

Garner administrative support

Administrators need to ensure that hospital systems are in place to support and foster good nurse-physician relationships. Organizations that don't provide affirmative and continuous administrative support should expect to fail, even in the face of Herculean efforts. Cooperation and collaboration start with the message sent by our leaders and by seeing the process in action.

In one area hospital, the SBAR tool failed due to lack of administrative support. Managers found a copy of the SBAR tool in their mailboxes, so they posted the flyer on their unit. Because it was delivered without any education or additional information, no one used the tool. Ideally, the SBAR tool should be introduced and discussed at medical staffing rounds and by nursing leadership.

Having a physician champion and a nurse champion who are dedicated to improving relationships is also critical to changing the culture. Another way to help change the culture is by engaging staff. Conducting a survey of staff satisfaction to determine the status of relationships on the unit or in your clinic is a good place to begin. In addition, joint educational projects and social events that build relationships are better attended when facilitated by administration. Administrators must work with physicians and nurses to identify trouble spots, develop plans, and implement strategies for building healthy relationships. From this level, the tone is set for physician-nurse relationships because behavioral standards, consequences, and zero-tolerance policies originate here.

On the unit level, the nurse manager must cultivate a collegial relationship with the chief of the department. This cohesive liaison serves as the ideal for physicians and nurses and establishes an atmosphere of solidarity. Only a collegial relationship with the medical counterpart is optimal for laying the groundwork for healthy nurse-physician partnerships. For example, nurse managers should send a weekly update to their medical counterparts (in easy-to-read bullet form) and plan regular monthly meetings. These meetings can be even more beneficial when incorporated into coffee or lunch.

Create a zero-tolerance policy

The Texas Nurses Association stepped forward and unanimously passed a resolution that called for zero tolerance of physician abuse. Verbal abuse is a broad category of behaviors that includes tone of voice and mannerisms. According to a 1999 survey conducted by registered nurses Araujo and Sofield, verbal abuse "leaves you feeling personally or professionally attacked, devalued, or humiliated." Further research indicated that 40% of nurses surveyed did not have a workplace policy that supported reporting of verbal abuse (Tabone, 2001).

A policy defines unacceptable behavior and its consequences, and it provides a much-needed support structure for nurses. However, a lone policy has proven not to be a deterrent to abuse unless it is followed and supported by both staff and administration. If your hospital or clinic has a policy, familiarize staff with it and cite specific examples of staff who have used this policy successfully. If there is no policy in place, advocate for one to be adopted—and that it be zero-tolerance.

In addition, the new Joint Commission standards mandate that all healthcare facilities have a policy to address disruptive behavior and conflict for their workplace (The Joint Commission, 2008). The standards require healthcare leaders to ensure a culture of safety and quality is created and maintained throughout the hospital. It also states that care can be harmed by disruptive behavior that intimidates staff or affects morale and staff turnover. The standards expect leaders to address the disruptive behavior of all individuals, no matter who they are or where they work, which includes clinical and administrative staff, management, licensed independent practitioners, and governing body members.

Provide assertiveness training

A policy alone is not sufficient. Staff must be given the skills and tools to address conflict, along with education about the new policy. A group of researchers led by Cook, Green, and Topp (2001) found that assertiveness training that focuses on conflict resolution and communication skills is an effective method of coping with verbal abuse. As another researcher, D. Buback (2004), says, "An assertive person informs the abuser of his or her feelings, letting the abuser know that the abuse will not be tolerated."

In Chapter 4, Mary exclaimed "No way!" when asked to stand up to her abuser—she did not have the assertiveness skills necessary to confront him. Like Mary, nurses are often hesitant to tell physicians to stop a behavior. They would benefit tremendously from learning assertiveness skills. Therefore, request hospital-based workshops or inservices. They teach such techniques as using short, specific statements that describe the event or behavior. They recommend that you say, for example, "Please do not yell. If you continue to yell, I will leave." Or, "I did not appreciate the comments you made in front of the patient today."

As Bubak (2004) writes, "Self-assertion is a method of learning about one's own limitations and strengths, which helps develop power and control."

Use your name as a powerful equalizer

Make sure that the physicians with whom you work frequently know your name. Daily communication should be mandatory—not optional—and calling someone by his or her name is a basic sign of respect. Therefore, introduce yourself to physicians, and if they forget your name, reintroduce yourself.

Always include something unique and personal about yourself or the person you are introducing (e.g., a hobby, your birthplace, etc.). When a physician can relate on a personal level, the relationship shifts; he stops viewing you as just another nurse and starts seeing you as a unique human being. Also, encourage new staff to wear a special nametag so that physicians can identify newcomers and make them feel welcome. This also gives physicians the "heads up" on staff who would benefit from receiving additional information.

Names can also shift a relationship from degrading to professional. At one hospital, a nurse approached me and asked whether there was anything specific she could do to improve a situation she was having with an older physician. The physician was not overtly abusive, but he was always subtly demeaning. My advice to her was that when there is a physician who is degrading and, as is often the case, he calls you by your first name, set the stage for a more equal relationship by saying, "I would appreciate it if you called me Mrs. _____, and not by my first name." Remember, names are powerful equalizers.

There was one physician who never did anything overt or raised his voice, but with his body language he consistently sent out the message that he was more important. So one day, I decided to even the playing field. I said, "Doctor, may I speak to you for a moment in private? I don't know how you started calling me by my first name when I call you by your last name. I would appreciate it if you called me Nurse Wakefield from now on as I call you Doctor Simmons."

He was surprised and readily agreed. But the next day, he couldn't remember my last name and, in frustration, said, "Barbara, please, just call me Jim."

"Certainly," I replied. And you should have seen the other nurses faces when I did!

Take advantage of formalized collaborative models

Collaborative governance models are based on building internal and external respect. They provide a structure for a working partnership that supports physicians and nurses both personally and professionally. (LeTourneau, 2004) suggests a model for collaborative practice in her article, "Physicians and Nurses: Friends or Foes?" First, the lead physician executive and the lead nurse executive must forge a collaborative and respectful relationship. In this way, they model the expected behavior for staff. The relationship they create is also a powerful message and symbol of partnership.

In order for this relationship to work, each party must understand the other's job. At one hospital, the chief nursing officer and the medical officer exchanged places for one day. The nursing officer followed a physician, and the medical officer followed a staff nurse.

At 10:00 a.m., the medical officer said emphatically, "We are never going to get this all done in one shift!"

"Oh yes we are," said the nurse as she proceeded at lightning speed with the organizational skills of a computer and the multitasking skills of an air traffic controller.

The physician commented on the remarkable speed and efficiency of the nurses. As a physician, he had written countless orders, but in his role as nurse, he now had to implement them. "I felt totally overwhelmed with the sheer number of details each nurse has to deal with on a daily basis," he remarked. It is an organizational challenge to administer a variety of medications to several patients at specific intervals.

Likewise, the chief nursing officer found the role of the resident—having to juggle operating time, round, and simultaneously answer calls and pages—a huge challenge (University of Washington News Rounds 11/3/2003). At the end of that day, their views of each other's reality had totally shifted, and the result was a powerful liaison.

Second, LeTourneau (2004) says, "the physician and nursing executives must initiate the development of an organizational vision of how physicians and nurses should work together for the benefit of the patient." Both groups should begin by identifying their expectation of the other group and of themselves.

Central to discussions of a shared vision, however, is a frank and open discussion and evaluation of how physician-nurse behavior affects the patient. Several of the true stories in this book are powerful testimonies. Therefore, one idea is to begin with true stories from your own unit—leaving out the names of those involved, of course.

Third, "the physician and nurse executives must lead their respective groups in translating the vision and expectations into behavior standards that apply to all and in establishing correction policies" (LeTourneau, 2004). Translating the vision in this way requires giving specific examples of how collaboration can be put into practice at your institution. For example, take the communication breakdowns on your unit, such as repetitive calls to a physician for a specific medication, and turn them into successes, such as standardized orders. Specific examples of nurses who are empowered to fulfill the vision and physicians who are committed to the vision are necessary in order for a new culture to take hold.

Build community

> *"Our core challenge is to create a mechanism by which we can have*
> *a meaningful sense of community, a discovery of core values,*
> *and a behavior change based upon the shared values" (Larson, 1999).*

Lecturer and writer Thomas Moore once said, "One of the greatest needs of the soul is for belonging." As the pace of life has increased over the past 50 years, membership in organizations, religious houses, and community activities has decreased by 45% (Putnam, 2000). Discretionary time has plummeted. Geographic mobility has resulted in many of us living miles away from our families, often our primary support systems. And despite rapid technological advances, economics dictate that we work harder than ever—most of us spend more time at work than we do at home. All of these factors make the workplace fertile common ground, where we have the potential to build meaningful relationships.

Although society places much value on technology and productivity, we are quickly learning that "social capital" is equally valuable. When we do not bond, retention is threatened and quality of care decreases with turnover. But if a nurse never has time to talk about her children or her life, she cannot bond with the group. If a physician does not indulge in the small talk that is the first step to connecting, then he will continue to feel like a stranger. Yet both nurses and physicians are working harder than ever. And because of this, some view the time we spend connecting with each other as extraneous or trivial. But it is not enough to recognize each other as professionals and simply perform the appropriate tasks. We must acknowledge each other as fellow human beings and connect by realizing that we are on the same journey.

Community is the optimal setting for bonding and, thus, patient safety. "Genuine community is a place where people feel safe to express themselves and to be themselves fully, without apology or explanation. The community offers acceptance" (Manion & Bartholomew, 2004). To form a safe working environment, the atmosphere on the unit must be psychologically safe. Fear of being judged or ridiculed is replaced by compassion, understanding, and belonging. Rather than trying to ignore the fact that we are human, both nurses and physicians acknowledge their humanness. Near misses and errors are reported in a blame-free zone with every member of the team owning their responsibility to "see it, own it, and say it." In such an environment, mistakes are anticipated, high-risk events rehearsed, and the expectation of perfection is left to robots.

In a community of people who genuinely care for each other, authority is decentralized—it is "a group of all leaders" (Manion & Bartholomew, 2004). The power differential that contributes significantly to unequal nurse-physician relationships is uprooted. When hierarchy disperses this way, individuals are valued for the areas in which they choose to lead. People are recognized for their unique contributions. For example, the nurse who fastidiously writes up quality discrepancies is respected for her constant vigilance—not criticized for her attention to details and policy. The physician who takes the lead on addressing infection or standardizing orders is valued for his time and energy. The nurse who makes us feel good and nourishes the work environment with her kindness and positive attitude is cherished, along with the doctor who consistently makes jokes. And when no one can place a difficult Foley catheter, everyone knows who to call. When staff are valued for their unique contributions, we raise the bar of our collective esteem. Liberation from oppression comes only after we become aware of what's happening and raise our self-esteem high enough that the oppression cannot possibly continue (Roberts, 2000).

Strategies for Collaborative Relationships

When I have a good working relationship with a physician, I feel comfortable approaching him or her, asking questions, and more respected for my own expertise. And the patient also benefits because they receive the best care.
—Lynsi Slind, University of Washington MSN student

Home runs!

Physician-nurse summit: Nurses began by surveying both physicians and nurses about what kind of relationship they wanted—and didn't make assumptions that collegiality was the goal for both. They then tabulated the responses and held a two-hour meeting where results were shared. This summit had both a physician and nurse champion and was held over dinner using a neutral facilitator. The primary focus was "What does each group need from the other in order to improve patient care?"

Improving emergency room MD-RN relationships: Both physicians and nurses were asked to make a list of the five things they wished each group would do that would affect patient care. After the list was compiled, both groups met for dinner and presented their top five things. Both groups were surprised and learned a lot about each other.

Source: TeamSTEPPS Project, Washington.

Enhancing education: Hot topics in critical care: A seminar was organized to update nurses in current critical care practice. A nurse and physician from each critical care unit collaborated to identify a current hot topic for their area of specialty from end-of-life issues to necrotizing fasciitis. Each dyad had one hour—the physician began with 30 minutes about the current state of the science, and then the nurse partner spoke on nursing assessment, intervention, and best practice.

Source: AACN National Teaching Institute, May 2006, Univ. of California, Irvine.

ICU joint practice: The ICU medical director and other physicians were invited to attend a portion of the unit staff meeting that dealt with operational, clinical, and quality issues. The meeting was co-facilitated by the nurse manager and medical director, and lunch was provided. Practices that would improve outcomes were identified and implemented. Both nurses and physicians offered examples of frustrating or disrespectful interactions and problem solving. Nurses and physicians enthusiastically report an increase in collaboration, subjective comfort, and confidence communication levels.

Source: AACN National Teaching Institute, May 2006, Unity Hospital, Minn.

Pediatric simulation: Using three mock codes with life-threatening scenarios, a set of standardized measures and observational techniques were used to determine nurse-physician collaboration. Although participants reported good collaboration each time, analysis of the tapes revealed that collaboration improved over time.

Read more: "Enhanced Nurse-Physician Collaboration Using Pediatric Simulation" by Patricia Messmer, PhD, RN, BC, FAAN.

Critical care nurse presentations during bedside rounds: Nurses were given a formal opportunity to provide the most recent information. Worksheets were developed to organize and reference information during the presentation. Residents presented assessment findings and diagnostic test results. Nursing staff at the SICU at Harborview Medical Center, WA, have verbalized an increase in overall job satisfaction and autonomy in their position.

Source: AACN National Teaching Institute, May 2006 abstract by Amy Stafford.

Out of the park: In New Hampshire, approximately 20 nurses, pharmacists, case managers, physicians, clinical coordinators, educators, and supervisors pulled together for Transforming Care at the Bedside (TCAB). The mission was to establish a patient-centered healing environment that was beneficial to all. Starting on a 28-bed telemetry unit, they first focused on their communication with each other and implemented bedside shift reporting, a daily safety huddle, and then "intentional" rounding. Intentional rounding means the nurse, doctor, and patient actively participate at the same time in a conversation about the patient's care. Physician-nurse satisfaction increased from 78% to 91%, and nurses report an increased feeling of collaboration and a sense of feeling valued. Even though this was rolled out on one unit, physicians now actively seek out nurses in other parts of the hospital. Kudos to staff who were dedicated to changing the culture in a project that spanned more than three years.

Read more: "Improving Communication Among Nurses, Patients, and Physicians" by Kimberly Chapman, MS, RN, CNL. American Journal of Nursing, Nov. 2009.

Addressing conflict and uniting under a zero-tolerance policy for disruptive behavior and verbal abuse is paramount. Yet there are many other strategies that a staff nurse can adopt as well to foster better communication and collaboration between nurses and physicians:

1. Understand that the difference in your roles may cause confusion. Reinforce your role in patient care. Use the progress notes to identify concisely the problems you addressed on your shift, the progress made, and the plan of care. Remember, be brief. Use SOAP (subject, observation, assessment, plan) charting.

2. Education is key to gaining knowledge and respect. Further your education in any way possible—from pursuing a bachelor's degree to pursuing a master's degree. Take advantage of certification courses in your specialty. Request assertiveness training workshops at your institution. Sponsor a conference by nurses and physicians. Turn physician complaints about nursing knowledge deficits into inservices. Use the vast knowledge of the experienced professionals around you to raise your level of knowledge.

3. Perform a root cause analysis whenever there is an unplanned outcome, and include both physicians and nurses on the team. Make harm visible and share the learning points with the team (Knox & Simpson, 2004; LeTourneau, 2004).

4. Ask for what you want. If you feel strongly that the physician needs to see a patient, say so. You don't have to have a diagnosis because you are not the doctor.

5. Communicate using the SBAR tool. When preparing your information prior to the phone call, remember that doctors want the facts to be fast, complete, and concise. Always be prepared to include your recommendation. If you are uncertain, review the case with your charge nurse or manager. Daily communication is required. Some people even use an additional D (SBARD), which stands for decision (Byrum, 2010).

6. Insist that physicians call you by name. Remind them if they forget.

 Speak Your Truth

7. Be prepared for telephone calls by having the chart, labs, and recent vital signs in your hand if there is a change in patient status.

8. Round with physicians whenever possible. If staffing is tight on the unit, take turns. There is no better way to learn what a physician is looking for, to clarify nursing's role, and to offer input.

9. Remind coworkers and physicians that you are all on the same team.

10. Advocate for the patient. Keep the patient as the main focus of conversation. Advocate for a formalized collaborative practice model.

11. Take personal responsibility for working out any negative relationships that you may have with a physician. Always take these conversations off the floor. Remember, "If you see it, you own it." Ask for manager support, if needed. Nurses report that they are often surprised that simply stating how a behavior makes them feel to a physician will heal the situation. Raising awareness of the problem and maintaining boundaries in this way is critical.

12. Connect with coworkers first. Promote a sense of belonging by forming a community of people who genuinely care about each other. Realize that nurses must have solidarity in order to raise their self-esteem. Then connect on a human level with the physicians. The work environment is a product of your relationships.

13. Acknowledge positive behavior and relationships. If there are physicians with whom you enjoy working, send thank-you notes and list specific reasons why you enjoy working with them. Send copies of the notes to the medical staffing office.

References

Araujo, Susan, and Laura Sofield (1999). "Verbal Abuse." *https://home.comcast.net/~laura08723/survey.htm* (accessed October 19, 2004).

Buback, D. (2004). "Assertiveness Training to Prevent Verbal Abuse in the OR." *Association of Operating Room Nurses* 79 (1).

Byrum, 3. (2010). "Convergent HR3." Lecture to VHA Southeast leaders on May 17, 2010,

Cook, J., M. Green, and R. Topp. (2001). "Exploring the Impact of Physician Verbal Abuse on Perioperative Nurses." *Association of Operating Room Nurses* (9): 317–331.

Copnell, B. (2003). "Doctors' and Nurses' Perceptions of Interdisciplinary Collaboration in the NICU, and the Impact of a Neonatal Nurse Practitioner Model." *Journal of Clinical Nursing* 13 (1): 105–113.

Elder, R., J. Price, and G. Williams. (2003). "Differences in Ethical Attitudes Between Registered Nurses and Medical Students." *Nursing Ethics* 10 (2): 149–161.

Ferrand, E., F. Lemaire, B. Regnier, et al. (2003). "Discrepancies Between Perceptions by Physicians and Nursing Staff of Intensive Care Unit End of Life Decisions." *American Journal of Resp. Critical Care Medicine* 67 (10): 1310–1315.

Greenfield, L. (1999). "Doctors and Nurses: A Troubled Partnership." *Annals of Surgery* 230 (3): 279–288.

The Joint Commission. (2008). "Behaviors That Undermine a Culture of Safety." *www.jointcommission.org/NewsRoom/PressKits/Behaviors+that+Undermine+a+Culture+of+Safety/app_stds.htm* (accessed April 2010).

Kingston, M., et al. (2004). "Attitudes of Doctors and Nurses Towards Incident Reporting: A Qualitative Analysis." *The Medical Journal of Australia* 181 (1): 36–39.

Knox, E., and K. Simpson (2004). "Teamwork: The Fundamental Building Block of High Reliability Organizations and Patient Safety." Workshop handout. Chicago: University of Chicago Safety Group.

Larson, E. (1999). "The Impact of Physician-Nurse Interaction on Patient Care." *Holistic Nursing Practice* 13 (2): 38–47.

Leonard, M., S. Graham, and D. Bonacum. (2004). "The Human Factor: The Critical Importance of Effective Teamwork and Communication in Providing Safe Care." *Quality and Safe Health Care* 13 (Suppl 1): 185–190.

LeTourneau, B. (2004). "Physicians and Nurses: Friends or Foes?" *Journal of Healthcare Management* 49 (1): 12–16.

Manion, J., and K. Bartholomew. (2004). "Community in the Workplace." *Journal of Nursing Administration* 34 (1).

Putnam, R. (2000). *Bowling Alone: The Collapse and Revival of American Community.* New York: Simon and Schuster.

Raica, D. (2009). "Effect of Action-Oriented Communication Training on Nurses' Communication Self Efficacy." *Med-Surg Nursing* Nov/Dec 2009.

Roberts, S.J. (2000). "Development of a Positive Professional Identity: Liberating Oneself From the Oppressor Within." *Advances in Nursing Science* 22 (4): 71–82.

Tucker. A.L, and S.J. Spear. (2006). "Operational Failures and Interruptions in Hospital Nursing." *Health Services Research* 41(3)(Pt 1): 643–662.

A Manager's Quest to Create Collegial Relationships

"Somebody has to do something, and it's incredibly pathetic that the somebody is us."
—Jerry Garcia, Grateful Dead

After three years on the neurology unit, I was becoming restless. One day a nurse from the orthopedic unit floated to our floor and told me about a new position: orthopedic supervisor. Not wanting to step on anyone's toes, I approached her gingerly to assess the opportunity better.

"Diane, I was thinking of applying for the supervisor position, and I wanted to know what you thought of the idea—wanted to make sure that it was okay with you," I said, realizing she was a key staff member.

"Are you kidding?" she replied. "That position had been open for over a year and a half. Why do you think it's still open? No one wants it!"

From the times I had floated over to the unit, I knew the orthopedic physicians could be pretty aloof. In fact, just last week I heard a rumor about how one of them had screamed at the manager in front of everyone. Still, as a nurse with only five years' experience, I wasn't making the money I needed. Maybe this was an opportunity in disguise—albeit a less than attractive disguise.

With no competition, I easily assumed the role as orthopedic supervisor (there wasn't anyone hanging around the bottom of this corporate ladder). I was incredibly naïve. Five months later, a massive reorganization put me first in line for the leading role of orthopedic manager. I could feel Fate's hand on my back, pushing me like a reluctant child onto the administration stage.

On my first Friday after taking the job, I greeted two of the orthopedic physicians in the hall. "Good morning, Dr. Winter. Good morning, Dr. Collins." I felt so small. How was I going to pull this off? I needed a costume or something—at least so I could fool myself. That weekend, I bought several suits and an extra long lab coat so that I would at least look different because I certainly didn't feel different in my new position. On some level, however, I knew that in order to change the culture, I had to improve the relationships. So as I headed to work that first day, I whistled my favorite song from the musical "The King and I" over and over again: "While shivering in my shoes, I strike a careless pose, I whistle a happy tune, and no one ever knows ... I'm afraid."

The Power of a Name

The clothes I had purchased had a transformational effect. They made me say things I would never dream of saying in a nurse's uniform. When Drs. Winter and Collins walked onto the floor that Monday, I spontaneously erupted, "Hi Jim! Hi Bob!" I didn't hang around long enough to see the looks on their faces. I hurried to my office, and as soon as the door shut, I breathed a deep sigh of relief. Was my Nordstrom personal shopper really my fairy godmother in disguise?

There was no reason to ever leave my office that first month; my first assignment was to complete 73 performance evaluations. At first I cursed my decision to take the job, but I slowly came to the realization that this was a great opportunity for me to get to know my staff.

One day, I was invited to a retirement party for a physician who had worked at the hospital for 30 years. The celebration was held at an art museum, and despite the open invitation, only about five nurses attended. Out of the corner of my eye, I could see Carrie standing alone by a painting, so I made my way across the room to talk with her. "After 15 years," she said, "they don't even know my name."

"What?" I replied. "What are you talking about?"

"I just walked by two of the physicians and realized they didn't know who I was. Fifteen years working full-time with these guys every day, and they don't even know my name," she said with saddened frustration. I was shocked.

As I made my way through the performance evaluations that month, I talked to staff and discovered that the vast majority were nameless like Carrie. Why would anyone want to work here, without the most basic of recognition?

When the evaluations were finished, it was time for me to meet with the physicians. Retention was my greatest challenge in a nursing shortage, and at the time, I had several open positions.

I needed to address an issue or two. Every Friday morning the physicians would gather in the One East conference room for rounds. They would present various x-rays and discuss among themselves the best approaches to difficult cases. One Friday, I cautiously approached the chief of orthopedics, who was chairing the meeting. "I need to speak to the doctors," I said. "I'd like to introduce myself, and I have a few important things I want to say." My heart felt like it was beating out of my chest as I waited for the first physician to finish his case. It was show time.

"My name is Kathleen Bartholomew, and I am the new manager of the orthopedic unit. Over the past month, I have had the opportunity to speak with every single staff member in order to finish their annual evaluations. Through these discussions, I learned that I have a serious problem. My number one problem is retention—and one of the biggest impediments to keeping staff is you. It simply is not possible to retain staff—or to have good working relationships with them—when you don't even know their names." I asked for their help. I had a plan.

Each Friday at "halftime," when one physician would take down his films and another set up his, I stood in front of the physicians brandishing a manila folder packed with information about a particular nurse. "This nurse," I began, "played the trumpet at Ronald Reagan's inaugural address. She loves gardening and has two cats. Her name is ..." I would follow this by pulling out an 8 x 10 picture of the nurse from the folder.

One by one, over the course of one year, I reintroduced staff to members who had worked with the physicians for years. "This nurse," I said one morning, "told me that she loved ballroom dancing and gardening, but when I dug a little deeper, I found out that she used to be a member of the Hell's Angels motorcycle club. Trading in her black leather jacket for whites, this is ..." I can recall instances when their curiosity would push them to the edges of their seats.

Not acknowledging someone's name is dehumanizing. This was most evident in colonial times, when it was common practice for masters to devalue their slaves by stripping them of their identity and referring to them as "boy" or "girl." By doing so, the owners were able to lump all slaves into a single category and dehumanize them.

Another example can be found in the book *Nickel and Dimed: On (Not) Getting By in America*. Its author, Barbara Ehrenreich, PhD, attempts to live on minimum wage for one year. The following is one of her earliest observations: "No one recognizes my face or my name, which goes unnoticed and for the most part unuttered. In this parallel universe where my father never got out of the mines and I never got through college, I am 'baby,' 'honey,' 'blondie,' and, most commonly, 'girl.'" Ehrenreich found that while working minimum-wage jobs, people did not find it necessary to use her name or know who she was—she was just a worker.

Likewise, not learning nurses' names allows physicians to lump us into a single group, rather than treat each of us as the sentient individuals we are. When we are nameless, it's easier for physicians—who form the dominant group—to justify using verbal abuse to remain in their superior positions.

Therefore, to form collaborative partnerships, physicians must know nurses' names. Acknowledging someone's name is the most basic and critical of all equalizers. The minute you have a name other than "nurse," the dynamics of the relationship will change.

Use Social Events as Networking Opportunities

By the time Christmas arrived, the atmosphere on the unit was much more cordial. One of the physicians kindly volunteered his home for a party—another chance to knit the fabric of this community closer together. I greeted each person who came through the door and handed him or her a nametag. I asked nurses, nursing assistants, and secretaries to write their first names on the tags. The physicians, however, were required to write down something interesting about themselves—a hobby, their most recent vacation, etc. One doctor wrote the school he went to, and I ripped it up. "We need something interesting," I explained. The tags were a wonderful way to melt the ice that froze a year of conversations that should have occurred but probably would not have otherwise.

As I watched the group interact, I realized the power of what was taking place. We were communicating as human beings, and the wall that usually separated us was being leveled by our common interests and our common humanity.

For example, after Sarah realized that she and Dr. Peters had children on the same soccer team, their relationship was never the same. When time permitted, they would talk as equals about their children's last game. The energy had changed, and telephone calls to Dr. Peters became a pleasure. They had found a way to connect and appreciate each other outside of the doctor-nurse realm.

The Great Fruit War: Conquering with Humor

And then there was the banana. Orthopedic physicians are not known for their creativity and spontaneity, so it was no surprise when Dr. Carrie entered the unit with a banana in his coat pocket—as he had done every day for the past three years. And like clockwork, he hung his coat on a chair (or the vacuum cleaner) and began making his rounds.

One day, however, the nurses decided to mix things up by writing a friendly message on the trusty banana. They took the banana out of Dr. Carrie's pocket and wrote on it, "Have a nice day!" They followed this good-natured act of mischief the next day by sticking in the other pocket of his coat an orange that read, "Orange you ready for a change?"

At 7:00 a.m. the next day, the joke was returned to the nurses when they discovered a large green apple on the counter of their station. On the apple, the doctor had written, "You guys are good to the core." That was the beginning of the "Great Fruit War," which is still going on today. In fact, this summer, "Christini the Zucchini" made her debut as a modern work of art—complete with medicine cup breasts and a gauze bikini. Her appearance pleased the good doctor and brought much-needed humor to the floor.

Nursing Through a New Lens

There were several other opportunities to elevate nursing in the eyes of the physicians—and the rest of the personnel at the hospital. After about five meetings with the spine physicians, which I had called to obtain much-needed information for a database, attendance began to dwindle. I learned that the spine physicians were reluctant to add another meeting to their calendars because they already met once a month at "Journal Club." For Journal Club, the physicians gathered at each others' homes to analyze and discuss articles assigned to each doctor. "Great!" I thought, and I asked a doctor for directions. It was almost humorous to see such surprise and disbelief awkwardly manifest itself on the typically unflappable doctor's face. He looked like I had asked him for the code to the doctors-only lounge.

As I walked up the long entryway to the house, I thought, "What am I doing here?" Soon after, I found that I was able to learn a great deal by simply listening; I fully appreciated the dialogue and even participated by offering information, when needed, about postop care. It was easy to see why these meetings were more desirable than mine—not to mention that they included beer and pizza.

One evening, after about four months, a physician turned to me and asked, "Kathleen, why don't you present next time?" I was thrilled at his suggestion, and I presented a master's level nursing paper on the effects of tissue oxygenation. Nurses were now being recognized as equal members of the patient-care team, and the collegiality that stemmed from these meetings was invaluable to all of the stakeholders.

A Meeting of the Minds

I established a place for myself at the Friday orthopedic rounds meeting. Introducing the nurses had given me a steady time slot, and I wasn't about to lose the only opportunity I had to speak with every physician. I used halftime to communicate problems and improvements on the unit, which initiated collaborative dialogue. The care pathways and patient education, which were more than 10 years old, were finally updated. Our shared vision of providing excellent quality care emerged, and physicians began to see the benefits of working together.

One Friday, the physicians requested point-of-care testing. I met with the person responsible for that program and invited her to present at the next "rounds," as it became known. Through our dialogue, we discovered that the root of the current problem, efficiency of patient care, was that physicians did not have their lab results when they rounded each morning.

To further hamper the process, nurses would get the results some time between 10:00 a.m. and 11:00 a.m.—when the physicians had already left the floor or hospital to perform a surgery or to see patients in their office. The nurse would then have to call the physician, who was busy caring for other patients. This was a huge interruption for both caregivers. Further, many physicians simply started writing blanket orders to avoid the interruption. A physician might order, "Give two units of blood if the hematocrit is below 29." Then, as Murphy's Law would dictate, the result would come back at 28.9. Not only did this system increase blood utilization, but it increased costs and labor.

I recall one physician's fantasy during a rounds session: "How about when I come to the floor at 7 a.m., there is a piece of paper waiting that lists all of my patients and their lab results?" Right. It was hard to keep a straight face. However, I dutifully put through a work order to the information services department. Much to my surprise, this one physician's fantasy became a reality.

After a few years, we broached the delicate arena of physician practices. There was great resistance because every physician believed his way was the best. How was I going to get them to move from ego-based practice to evidence-based practice? If I walked into rounds and asked for standardization, no physician would listen. It took me weeks to come up with a solution.

Creative strategies

One Friday, I asked the physicians to watch my "New Nurse Orientation Film." I explained that it was less than 15 minutes long and that all I needed was for them to imagine themselves as a new nurse arriving on our unit for training. The PowerPoint presentation began with posterior precautions for hip patients—and suddenly a name flew in from the right, onto the screen. These, apparently, were Dr. Jordan's precautions. There were two more slides of posterior precautions—all with individual names attached.

I then moved onto dressing changes and listed every doctor's specific instructions. Some insisted on cutting the steri-strips in half, some wanted a Band-Aid® dressing, etc. By the time the sixth slide came into view, they were squirming in their seats. I had used a digital camera to take a picture of the white board in the conference room, which gave extremely detailed instructions from one surgeon: "Do not use toppers, use 4 x 4 sponges, etc." I listed which doctors said you could shower patients on postop days four or five and which said you couldn't. I listed the doctors whose drain you could pull and whose you could not.

At the end of the presentation, I said, "Now, you are a new nurse with six patients and at least four different doctors. I hope you can remember which doctor will let their patient shower on the third day and which physician likes their steri-strips cut in half." Judging by the looks on their faces, it was clear that the physicians had never before seen their requests from this point of view. The physicians voted to standardize their practices, with only two requests: start with the easiest, and bring one practice at a time to their attention. We are now on the fourth slide and continue plugging along.

Educational Opportunities

Last year, three of the staff nurses decided to bring back the Annual Educational Conference—an event that had not been held in years. Historically, the conference would draw nurses from a five-state region, and the turnout would elevate their collective self-esteem. The nurses worked diligently with a handful of physicians who volunteered to speak, and they designed an outstanding all-day program. The event put the hospital on the map and gave the nurses and physicians the common goal of being the regional center for expertise in their field.

Enhancing joint educational opportunities is an excellent way to build nurse-physician relationships because it closes the vast educational gap. Because physicians are equally pressured for time, informal and impromptu inservices work best. Physicians are encouraged to come in after report and speak about specific areas of concern.

For example, there was a surgeon who wanted staff to be alerted to particular symptoms during postoperative care, so he gave a 15-minute talk about two cases in which he was not notified in a timely manner, thereby causing adverse patient outcomes. He actively encouraged nurses to call him for concerns related to these symptoms.

Just What the Doctor Ordered: A Physician's Prescription for Transforming Our Culture

by Jon Burroughs, MD, MBA, FACPE, CMSL

How can we rebuild a culture that has taken so long to evolve and that seems to permeate everything we do, feel, think, and say?

First, we cannot do it alone or within the isolation of our respective professional silos. It is true that only a nurse can understand another nurse or that only a physician can understand another physician from a professional point of view. And yet, this historic separation is a major part of the problem that we must remove by carefully and respectfully taking down the professional barriers that separate us. This can be done in part through the following ways:

1. **Education for both physicians and nurses.** For physicians, we need to be re-educated in how to work in teams with other healthcare professionals in an interdisciplinary and interdependent way, to learn from each other, support each other in our complementary duties, and to respect and appreciate one another. For nurses, the two-year vocational educational system needs to be replaced by a professional program that prepares nurses to deal with 21st century technology and equips them with knowledge and a seat at the professional table. Equality must be earned, and tens of thousands of nurses are pursuing bachelor's, master's, and doctorate-level programs that place them on an intellectual par with their physician colleagues. The nursing educational system has unwittingly

established and sustained the self-inflicted and destructive indentured servitude of the nursing profession, and it must end.

2. **Communication.** Kathleen has emphasized this point throughout the book. Three concrete ways to improve physician-nursing communication are to create a physician-nursing council, hold an annual physician-nursing summit, and initiate intentional or interdisciplinary rounds daily, with monthly grand rounds.

   • A physician-nursing council is often made up of medical staff and nursing leaders along with the CEO and a representative of the governing board's executive committee. The purpose of this council is to develop a basis for intercollegial dialogue regarding global issues that have a direct and indirect effect upon patient care, patient safety, and the achievement of important quality and financial goals. Policies and procedures may be developed as well as overall approaches to interdisciplinary care. Serious behavioral issues may be collaboratively discussed so that all are in agreement about how they will be managed by an interdisciplinary leadership team.

   • A physician-nursing summit is an excellent opportunity for each group to speak their truths and to appreciatively listen to the other. In addition, important agreements around care, communication, and overarching protocols may be established. For example, at a recent physician-nursing summit, the physicians agreed on zero tolerance for disruptive behavior and agreed to hold themselves accountable to eliminate such destructive communication. In return, nurses agreed not to over-populate the night shift with inexperienced new graduates, to universally utilize SBAR by the most experienced nurse present, and to eliminate nonurgent telephone calls throughout the night. These conferences can be a "win-win" and go a long way to reestablishing mutual trust, understanding, and respect.

• Intentional or interdisciplinary rounds represent the future of healthcare. Solo rounds are silo rounds in which little communication takes place between caregivers, redundant non-value-added work is done, discharge planning and case management grind to a halt, and medical errors unintentionally occur. Traditional weekend rounds are even worse, with little advancement in care, little if any case management (we do traditional case management during banking hours and wonder why our lengths of stay are too long), and things falling through the cracks. Ideally, nurses and physicians should coordinate their schedules so that rounding never interferes, but rather complements the change-of-shift routine so that all key caregivers can participate in a meaningful way. This may require some flexibility and dedication to the principle that intentional rounds and the opportunity to communicate directly with all key practitioners should take precedence over traditional schedules.

'Aunt Jane'

In *Uncle Tom's Cabin*, Harriet Beecher Stowe wrote about the plight of American slaves. She tells how Uncle Tom courageously led slaves to freedom via the Underground Railroad. To outline the courage needed to make change within hospitals and pull nurses up so they can function on a collegial level with physicians, S. Roberts draws similarities between Uncle Tom and the nurse's best advocate—the nurse manager—in his article, "Development of a Positive Professional Identity: Liberating Oneself From the Oppressor Within" (2000). Those nurses, staff, or management who lead the way out of oppression are, he says, Aunt Janes.

Charge nurses and nurse managers are in an opportune position to change the culture of nurse-physician relationships. They are at the front lines, where the action is happening. It takes courage and timely intervention to affect nurse-physician relationships on the unit.

Recently I spoke at a nursing conference. There are few statistics about supervisors who witness verbal abuse, so during my presentation, I asked the audience how many managers had witnessed disruptive behavior. Three-quarters of the audience raised their hands. One of the common tenets of any service excellence program is, "If you see it, you own it." In other words, if you witnessed the abuse, then you have an obligation to draw attention to it so that it doesn't happen again.

But nurse managers do not take ownership of this problem—many go out of their way to keep things smooth on the floor. In the meantime, however, simply standing by and doing nothing is passive acceptance of the situation, and diffusing conflict is yet another way in which we do not speak our truth. Every time we say and do nothing when a fellow nurse is being intimidated by a physician, we are just as responsible as he is.

And here it comes again, the rotating door of a question: Do we give our power away because we have been oppressed, or are we oppressed because we have given our power away? Either way, what is important is that we now recognize and acknowledge the moments when we feel small and powerless and that we respond differently. Our voice is our power. When involved in distressing interaction with a physician, many nurses lose their voice. The most common reason is that past experiences have left us burned. Sometimes it's because we lack the conflict management skills needed to handle confrontation. Another reason is that being silent is a characteristic of an oppressed group. And it only takes a few incidents of feeling insubordinate and insignificant to never speak again.

Lucille found the manager in her office. "Can I talk to you?" she asked hesitantly.

"Sure," said the manager. "What's going on?"

"Yesterday, Dr. Wyte came into a patient's room where I was working, and by the time he left I felt completely stupid. He belittled me in front of the patient, talking in a tone that was so condescending that I can't seem to pick myself up."

"Can you say something to him?" the manager asked.

Eyes downcast, Lucille mumbled, "No. I just can't."

There is no greater need in nursing management than for leaders to take a stand on physician-nurse relationships. Staff nurses desperately need—and deserve—leaders who will set the expectation for collegial relationships on the unit. The manager sets the standard and provides a model by her reactions to these incidents.

Staff ache for the words to articulate their stance, but they lack the language. Nursing leaders can model this voice and tell the truth about the effects these poor relationships have on our profession. The bottom line is that collegial relationships are an expectation set by the nurse manager.

Setting the standard

Yesterday, the patient in 960 went downhill fast—and hard. Pam had called the doctor to notify him that Mrs. Cally had increased shortness of breath, increased chest pressure, and decreasing oxygen saturations to the low 80s, requiring that the oxygen be turned up to four liters. But because the patient had a history of anxiety, the doctor said that he "wasn't worried." His only order was to continue monitoring the patient. But the patient kept calling out, "Help me. Help me," as she struggled to breathe—and the worried staff monitored her vital signs and tried to make her comfortable. Within an hour, her condition had deteriorated even further, and the nurse called the doctor again emphatically stating that this patient needed to be seen immediately. The doctor told his office nurse to relay the message that he would be over "within the hour." But Mrs. Cally didn't have an hour—and every nurse on the floor knew it.

Moral distress. Never in 27 years of nursing had Pam felt so helpless. Tears filled her eyes as she paged the manager. Ignoring the fact that there was no doctor's order, the charge nurse called the hospitalist stat as staff rushed the crash cart to the room. Luckily for Mrs. Cally, help arrived just in time. Her blood pressure plummeted as her saturations dropped to the 60s. The hospitalist gave stat orders and transferred the patient to the ICU, and the manager called the attending physician to tell him where he could now find his patient.

As the manager walked into the ICU, she heard the attending say to the hospitalist, "I guess I really should have listened to the nurses." Taking the attending off to the side, the manager then asked the physician if he could please go upstairs and "talk to the nurses ... because they did not feel heard." The manager then went to the phone and called the charge nurse and asked that, when the doctor arrived, the conversation be taken off the floor and into the conference room. She encouraged staff to speak honestly about how exasperated and helpless they had felt. In addition, she prompted them to ask the doctor if there was something else the nurses could have said that would have alerted him to the seriousness of the situation, thereby emphasizing both parties' roles in communication.

The doctor apologized for his lack of trust in the nurses' assessment. There was a tremendous amount of healing that happened that day—and a tremendous amount of respect for the doctor who had the courage to follow through, taking the time to validate the nurses' perceptions and honor their feelings.

Imagine that a nurse has come to you complaining about a physician who talked to her rudely and arrogantly. The nurse feels humiliated. The very next day, you see this physician on the unit. What do you do?

The day after Lucille spoke with the manager, Dr. Wyte came to the floor, and the secretary paged the manager regarding his arrival. "Dr. Wyte," the manager said, "can I talk to you for just a minute?" He nodded, and she opened the conference room door. "I understand that you had an interaction with Lucille yesterday that left her feeling devalued and insignificant."

He paused for a moment and then said, "I'm sorry. Will you tell her I'm sorry?"

"It would be better if you told her yourself," suggested the manager. "She is just down the hall."

     Speak Your Truth

Few professionals—not even busy physicians—will refuse a minute of their time. Perhaps that's why asking, "Can I talk to you for just a minute?" was well received by Dr. Wyte. There are other things you should do to ensure that such conversations go smoothly:

- Find a private place (e.g., a conference room) where you can sit down.

- Always take potentially emotional conversations off the floor.

- Make excellent eye contact and be direct.

- State what you know, and never judge the situation. For instance, if you say, "Excuse me, I understand that yesterday you had an interaction with one of my nurses that left her feeling devalued and unappreciated," you avoid direct accusation.

In this case, the doctor apologized but then asked the manager to "please apologize to the nurse for him." Don't accept the job as emissary of apologies. The standard of etiquette for apologizing was set in kindergarten—apologies are given directly to the person who has been offended by the offender.

By her actions, this manager demonstrated to both physicians and nurses the standard of acceptable behavior on the unit. Two-thirds of hospitals have approved standards detailing acceptable behavior, but nurses continue to report disruptive behavior in these institutions and do not find the standards to be helpful because they are not enforced. Therefore, although it is an excellent idea to lobby for behavioral standards, standards alone do not stop disruptive behavior—they are only as valuable as the nurses who use them.

Role modeling

> *Martina was charting at the nurses' station when a doctor came up to the desk and started yelling at her, "How many times do I have to tell you?" He was wildly shaking his finger in her face.*
>
> *Martina stood up and said, "Can I see you for a minute right now?" He answered by following her into the soiled utility room. Martina was very direct. "First of all," she said, "I am very smart, and if you tell me something once I will remember. I have no idea what you are yelling about. And second," she said, looking him directly in the eye, "don't ever wave your finger in my face like that again."*

When called on his behavior, the physician apologized. Fifteen minutes later, he came up to the desk and apologized again.

It is vital that nurse managers role model zero tolerance for any kind of disruptive, intimidating, or verbally abusive behavior. In order to support this standard, however, you—the nurse manager—also need support. The way to do so is to develop a close working relationship with the chair of your department. Doing so sets the tone for collegiality on the unit, and some issues are better handled peer to peer.

Remember, however, that you don't have to personally fix every situation to be effective. Managers must take action, but certain types of behavior and situation may call for indirect intervention.

> *Dr. David had been on the floor for less than a year. His relationship with the nurses began cordially enough, but after a while, the nurses became annoyed. Maggie was standing outside the patient's room when Dr. David wrote his orders. "Good thing I'm standing right here," she said, "because no one is going to be able to read your handwriting." The manager was making rounds and overheard the conversation. She glanced at the chart and heard the doctor say, "Yeah, I get written up every month for illegible handwriting."*
>
> *His whole manner was arrogant, and he clearly had no intention of trying to improve his handwriting.*
>
> *The next week, nurses reported that they had called Dr. David several times after 5 p.m. and that his responses were rude. That same day, the manager got a call in her office from the evening shift nurse taking care of one of Dr. David's patients. She had called the doctor and reported a dislocated hip, and he had not even bothered to come in and look at the patient.*

It's more difficult to deal with several occurrences that happen within a short period of time than it is to deal with one. In this case, the manager wrote a memo detailing the behavior to the chief of the department and peer review. Within a week, Dr. David came to the manager's office. He explained that personal events had been overbearing in his life at the time, and he apologized. Further, he emphasized that it would not happen again.

Aunt Jane's Top Tips for Managers

The manager (or charge nurse) is in a key position to improve nurse-physician relationships on the unit. A manager's response to disruptive behavior sets the standard for the unit— just as a lack of response also sets a standard. Hospital standards and policies are inefficient in and of themselves. Managers are present on the floor, at the front lines, where disruptive behavior and verbal abuse take place. Staff desperately need to see a zero-tolerance approach to disruptive behavior role modeled and enforced by their nurse managers. Therefore, from one Aunt Jane (nurse manager) to another, take the following actions to show your nurses that disruptive behavior will not be tolerated:

Create a shared vision:

- Find a physician champion

- Hold 100% of both nurses and physicians accountable for demonstrating professionalism at all times

- Survey both nurses and staff on satisfaction with each other—address issues openly

Develop strong relationships with your physician counterparts:

- Share a cup of coffee—get to know each other as professionals and human beings

- Ask, "How can nursing improve patient outcomes?" and "What can we do together to improve RN-MD relationships on the unit?"

- Keep physicians informed on recruitment and retention statistics

- Share process improvement goals and outcomes

- Write a thank-you note to a collegial physician every month

Set the standard for nurse-physician communication:

- Send weekly e-mails in bullet form to your physician counterpart/department chair

- Schedule a quarterly meeting

 Speak Your Truth

Aunt Jane's Top Tips for Managers (cont.)

Role model effective confrontation:

- Intervene immediately when you see/hear about disruptive behavior
- Be present and available on the floor during rounding
- Follow a different physician each week (for one day) on rounds

Insist that physicians call staff by name:

- Pair a new staff member with a physician mentor
- Use a different nametag (e.g., green border) for new staff

Organize joint educational events:

- Have a nurse and physician pair to work on a project or seminar

Organize social events as networking opportunities:

- Celebrate accomplishments
- Have participants wear nametags describing favorite hobby, etc.

Elevate nursing by presenting papers or best practice on clinical issues:

- Champion standardization and physician-nurse driven protocols

Invent creative strategies to nurture partnerships:

- Advocate for "intentional rounding"
- Set the expectation that a physician and nurse communicate face to face daily
- Facilitate post-procedure briefings whenever plan of care diverges from expected outcomes

Conclusion: Not So 'Pleasantville'

In the film *Pleasantville*, everything is black and white. The movie depicts the 1950s to the point of hyperbole: The characters all did exactly what they were supposed to do because they all inherently knew the rules. Without exception, the actors followed the same daily routine down to the smallest detail.

For years, our interactions with physicians have been just like that black-and-white drama. Everyone knows their part, and many of our responses are as rehearsed as a motion picture script. Few admit that there is a certain degree of comfort and security in knowing our lines—and few admit the challenge and difficulty of learning a new script. It's not easy to be impromptu, especially when the physician gives no indication of wanting to engage or is disruptive. But there are compelling reasons that beg for a rewrite, the greatest of which is the fact that every story in this book is true.

These tales are from the front line. There is nothing as powerful as the stories themselves. The patient did wait four hours in pain because the nurse was too intimidated to call the physician at night. The nurse was so upset by the physician's hostility that she fled to the bathroom with a nosebleed. And further, every nurse reading this book has a story of his or her own.

In *Pleasantville*, the main character gets sucked into a television sitcom and brings color to a previously dull and drab existence when she breaks from the "approved" script and kisses a boy. A rose suddenly changes from gray to vibrant red. Likewise, the quality of our relationships and the degree to which we care for each other adds color and life to what is ordinarily dull and gray—especially when we break from the script. It's the nurse who wrote on the banana and put it back in the physician's pocket and the doctor who exclaimed, "Good call!" to a nurse who offered a successful care solution who add meaning to our day. The quality of our relationships paints the atmosphere in which we work. By connecting with each other and celebrating our profession, and by changing the environment so that everyone in it is respected, acknowledged, and cared for, we can create the optimal environment for patients to heal and for nurses and physicians to work together.

References

Ehrenreich, Barbara. (2001). *Nickel and Dimed: On (Not) Getting By in America.* New York: Henry Holt and Company.

Roberts, S. (2000). "Development of a Positive Professional Identity: Liberating Oneself From the Oppressor Within." *Advances in Nursing Science* 22 (4): 71–82.

7

Leadership's Role: Creating and Sustaining Healthy Nurse-Physician Relationships

LEARNING OBJECTIVES

After reading this chapter, the participant will be able to:

- Describe leadership's role in creating and sustaining healthy nurse-physician relationships

- Discuss strategies leaders can use to deal with disruptive behavior

One Friday morning during rush hour, on January 12, 2007, a violinist set himself up at the L'Enfant Plaza Metro station in Washington, DC, and began to play several Bach pieces. After 43 minutes, five classical pieces, and 1,097 people passing by, he had collected only $32.17—even though the night before, this very same violinist, Joshua Bell, had commanded $100 a ticket playing on the very same Stradivarius.

The experiment, conducted by The Washington Post, *demonstrated that perception is greatly influenced by the setting. We see what we expect or want to see. In a subway, people expected to see a street musician, not a world-class virtuoso. Not only did they not see him, they didn't hear the music either.*

Likewise, perception of anomalies in our everyday setting is just as rare because we are continuously immersed in the setting.

Perceptions vs. Reality

Traveling around the country offers opportunities to observe how organizations have succeeded or failed at improving physician-nurse relationships. Seldom do I find hospitals that consider improving these relationships a priority initiative backed by a well-informed board of directors. Consistently, I encounter well-meaning leaders whose assessment of their own nurse-physician culture is off the mark because "individuals selectively see what reinforces their preexisting biases while failing to see what challenges those perceptions" (Bujak, 2008).

Research supports this observation. For example, perceptions of patient safety differ as we travel up the hierarchy: the view from the bedside doesn't match physician or administration's assessment (Buerhaus, 2007). Perceptions determine our reality. And the reality today is that nurse-physician relationships are far from optimal, while most leaders remain unaware of both the effect and frequency of disruptive behavior. But without administrative support, relationships will never significantly improve.

"The physician–nurse scores were in the low 90s, so administration was pleased. They don't realize that as long as everybody plays their status quo roles, things will be fine. On Monday, the charge nurse said to the doctor, "You owe me. I wrote orders for you all weekend." And the doctor responded, "You're the best, Karen!" and gave her a pat on the back. Physicians encourage nurses to practice beyond their scope.

Another doctor didn't want the nurse to tell the patient about an error, so he gently cajoled her saying, 'I need to know that you are with me on this one … there's nothing to be gained by telling the patient that we started to operate on the wrong side.' Sure, the scores are good. But you never asked why—and I could have told you."

—Surgical unit manager

****

> *"I get a visceral feeling in my gut whenever that physician comes to the floor. We stopped reporting his behavior years ago because nothing ever happens anyway."*
>
> *–Pediatric ICU RN*
>
> ************
>
> *"Last year, I had a consultant talk to my nurses and managers about understanding and improving MD-RN relationships. Then yesterday, I did a survey, and my directors listed MD-RN relationships as one of their top three problems. I can't believe it! This was the director level!"*
>
> *–CNO*

The greatest impediment to patient safety is culture. The reality is that the current health-care culture is one of avoidance and silence, and this culture can only be changed through strong leadership. Conflict avoidance is prevalent, along with a passive-aggressive communication style; we tell everyone but the person actually involved why we are upset. The Silence Kills studies (*www.silencekills.com*) confirm we avoid confrontation even when we see incompetence. Furthermore, when confronted, many physicians are unaware of their behavior and how they come across and are genuinely surprised at the feedback.

When stressed, all human beings revert unconsciously to earlier learned patterns of coping. By having the courage to have a conversation, we demonstrate caring and uphold the mission and values of our institutions. Ignoring this opportunity allows a single event to become routine. Every time leadership ignores a deviance, they inadvertently create a new norm.

The vast majority of these organizations already have a code of conduct policy—it's just not enforced. The greatest system factor that contributes to disruptive behavior is the culture of an organization. In a survey of 1,627 physician executives, 71% indicated that a code of conduct was already in place. Yet in this same group, 56.5% indicated that problem behaviors from physicians resulted in conflict between nurses or other staff (Weber). Administration follows a consistent pattern of tolerating the behavior of a few rogue physicians because they are good clinicians. Addressing the behavior of these disruptive physicians in the past often resulted in "I'll take my business elsewhere" and a significant financial loss for the organization, which set in place a pattern of tolerating the behavior for years. Hickson reminds us that "Unprofessional behavior begets more unprofessional behavior, especially if disruptive providers have 'protectors' or 'enablers' … providing administrative cover" (2007).

> *"I don't understand. How can you let this physician swear repeatedly at the nurses? What would you do if someone talked to your wife or daughter like that? And why do you hesitate to pass a red rule or code stating that all physicians must speak English? The same language is the most basic of requirements for patient safety."*
>
> —Consultant to CEO

Another way the structure of these organizations is designed for failure is because the medical director is set up to be the frontman and the main person responsible for dealing with disruptive physicians. Many medical directors say they feel impotent handling peer behavioral issues because they don't have any real—or even any perceived—power. They can't suspend or fire their colleagues. In addition, they aren't prepared to handle conflict, which makes them nervous because they have not been given the tools to handle these delicate situations that historically end up backfiring on them. Suddenly, they are the bad guy and have to pay the price for breaking the cultural code of professional omerta, which says, "I'll cover your back if you watch mine."

> *"Last time I intervened, I ended up wishing I had kept my mouth shut. My patient referrals dropped drastically. I was made to feel like I betrayed my peers just because I held the line. I can't afford to do that again."*
>
> —*Medical director*

The Joint Commission Sentinel Event Alert, "Behaviors that undermine a culture of safety," validates the current healthcare culture and its history of indifference. This alert acknowledges that institutions have failed to address disruptive behaviors on both the individual and system level, despite the known effect on patient care. Ignoring disruptive behaviors is no longer an option. The new Joint Commission standards clearly state organizations must manage conflict (LD 2.40) and healthcare leaders must "create and maintain a culture of safety and quality throughout the hospital" (LD 3.10).

Unfortunately, many institutions believe they have met Joint Commission standards so long as a code of conduct is in place. Although a code of conduct lays a critical foundation, it will fail if it is the sole intervention taken to address behavioral issues. Creating healthy nurse-physician relationships requires a sustained commitment to creating and supporting both the structure and processes necessary to address individual conflict. Significant improvements in physician-nurse relationships require total systemic cultural change and strong leadership.

Individual Response: One Bad Apple . . .

Even though fewer than 5% of physicians are disruptive, damage caused by this small group is exponential. It is not possible to create healthy teams if there is an exception to the rule, as this exception always and inevitably undermines the very foundation of teamwork, which is trust. A mission statement with sub-clauses and exceptions is no longer a mission statement. Institutional integrity can only be realized if and when the same standards apply to all; when the behaviors and language of all the employees in the organization consistently match the mission. Any culture or system that tolerates disruptive behavior has, in essence, approved a new behavioral norm.

Nurses react to this behavioral norm in certain ways. According to the Advisory Board, 30.7% leave the hospital; 24% refuse to work with a physician or change their schedule. Another study found that 30% of administrators, nurses, and physicians could name a nurse who left in the last year specifically because of a poor interaction (Rosenstein). Nurses are known to "self-silence" and have consistently demonstrated a lack of self-efficacy. Not only do they typically tolerate unprofessional behavior, they fail to report it because "that's just the way it is."

The erroneous belief that sustains organization's tolerance of disruptive behavior is that it's just "one bad apple." This couldn't be further from the truth. The effects of a single individual's negativity are exponential. Research shows that a single toxic team member is strongly linked with group level dysfunction. Negative individuals have an "asymmetric and deleterious effect on others" (Felps, 2006). As it turns out, how low the lowest team member scores on conscientiousness, agreeableness, and emotional stability is usually a strong predictor of group cohesion and the group's performance (Neuman & Wright). "You're only as strong as your weakest link" is an age-old adage now backed by research. Over time, individual reactions become group dysfunction.

Furthermore, negative events produce "larger, more consistent, and long-lasting effects as compared to positive thoughts, feelings, and events ... the 'bad apple is stronger than good phenomenon' " (Felps). So even though an institution has reached commendable quality and safety benchmarks, one negative employee can have an inordinately greater influence. In studies predicting marital success or divorce, for example, negative interactions are a more predictive factor than positive interactions (Felps).

What is known about these disruptive or "high conflict personalities" (Eddy, 2003)? They are high achievers and usually very good clinicians who have an inability to self-reflect. Rather than single events, they demonstrate enduring patterns of behavior. When confronted, they try to change the situation around or blame others and chronically identify as a helpless victim (Eddy). Because of the following reasons, they have often gotten away with their behavior for years.

Reasons why responses to disruptive behavior have been ineffective:

- Unclear/no expectations for conduct

- Professional conduct expectations not modeled by leadership or faculty

- Inconsistent application of policy/infrequent enforcement

- Response is late—occurs after a serious event

- Narrow process options force delay—fear of escalation

- Approaches address the individual only and not the system or culture

- Poor conflict engagement skills—failure to engage (Gerardi, 2008)

Process for Guiding Interventions

The "Disruptive behavior pyramid" (Figure 3) developed by Dr. Gerald Hickson and his colleagues at Vanderbilt University School of Medicine provides an excellent visual framework for dealing with disruptive physicians (or nurses, or any member of the healthcare team). This framework serves as a foundation for training staff on how to provide feedback. As reflected in the pyramid, the vast majority of physicians consistently exhibit professional behavior, and disruptive physicians are the tip of the iceberg. Metaphorically, however, these disruptive physicians are the barrier we hit that will sink our organizational ships no matter how wonderful we think we are.

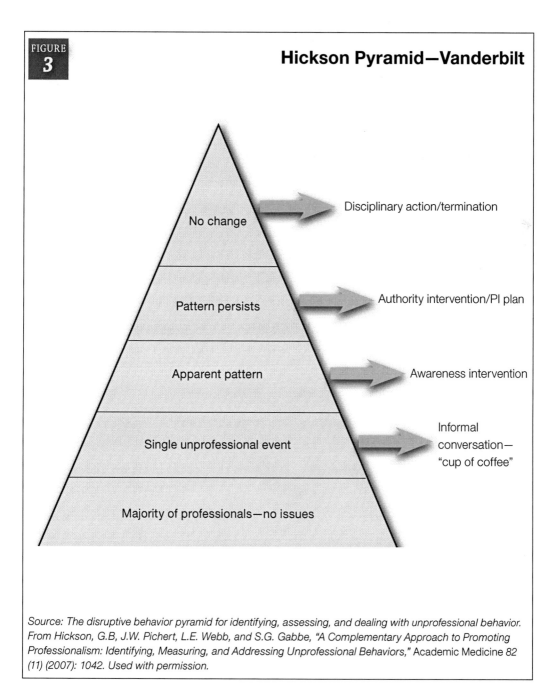

FIGURE 3

Hickson Pyramid—Vanderbilt

No change → Disciplinary action/termination

Pattern persists → Authority intervention/PI plan

Apparent pattern → Awareness intervention

Single unprofessional event → Informal conversation— "cup of coffee"

Majority of professionals—no issues

Source: The disruptive behavior pyramid for identifying, assessing, and dealing with unprofessional behavior. From Hickson, G.B, J.W. Pichert, L.E. Webb, and S.G. Gabbe, "A Complementary Approach to Promoting Professionalism: Identifying, Measuring, and Addressing Unprofessional Behaviors," Academic Medicine 82 (11) (2007): 1042. Used with permission.

The following strategies are based on Hickson et al.'s model.

Single unprofessional incident

Any type of disruptive behavior is not normal. Behaviors and remarks both overt and covert that do not contribute to the synergy and well-being of the team are unprofessional. Furthermore, it is the *perception* of unprofessionalism that warrants a conversation, so that together you can share your individual realities and reach the common ground critical for collegial teamwork.

A typical reaction when a disruptive physician is confronted about his or her behavior is that the physician will use a systemic problem as an excuse. For example, "The nurse should have known better. The MRI wasn't read for over two hours." There are two issues here: the behavior and the system problem, but the system problem is not an excuse. Be careful to address each issue separately. There is never a rationale for disruptive or unprofessional behavior.

Single incidents warrant a 'cup of coffee' conversation that should be carried out as soon as possible after the incident. The cup of coffee, if possible, should be done in a private setting, should involve a single event only, is never therapeutic in nature, and is delivered with the notion that the observation could be wrong (for example, "I saw, heard, or witnessed, but I could be wrong"). The informal conversation generally lasts only a couple of minutes and may be used by any member of the healthcare team, such as nurse-to-physician, nurse-to-nurse, or physician-to-nurse.

NOTE: Exceptions to this informal intervention are rule breaking such as substance abuse, allegations of sexual boundary violations, and suspicions of impaired practice, which all require immediate reporting (Hickson).

Apparent pattern of behavior

If unprofessional or disruptive behavior recurs and a persistent pattern of behavior emerges, an 'awareness intervention' is conducted by an authority figure or a peer-trained messenger. Choose a private setting and share pertinent data, such as graphic displays, peer-based data comparisons, or an individual complaint report. Then pause to allow the individual an opportunity to respond. Invite the other person's viewpoint and encourage the person to reflect on the event and why he or she seems to be associated with more events than other members of the group. Avoid diagnoses or prescriptions and encourage creative problem solving. If possible, always follow with expressing appreciation for the person's individual contribution to the team (Hickson).

Authority intervention

Failure to respond to an awareness intervention results in an authority intervention. This type of intervention requires leaders to develop improvement and evaluation plans for continued accountability. The plan is tailored to the extent and severity of the issue and may include a review of practice systems or protocols, health evaluation, or relevant continuing medical education training. The acronym for the authority intervention is EDICTS:

Expectations
Deficiencies
Intervention
Consequences
Timeline
Surveillance

Disciplinary intervention

Failure to respond to an authority intervention results in disciplinary action. This is the tip of the pyramid and requires restriction or termination of privileges with appropriate reporting to government entities (Hickson).

In one institution, the authority intervention stage requires the physician to attend a series of individual counseling sessions that cost the physician $6,000 out of his or her own pocket. After one year, if there are no subsequent patient or staff complaints about the physician, the hospital reimburses the fee.

System Response: . . . Spoils the Whole Bunch

This above process for addressing individual physician behavior must include simultaneous supporting actions to create healthy nurse-physician collaborative partnerships. A code of conduct means nothing without interventions, which will fail if staff are not adequately trained on how to respond to conflict. And even codes and skilled interventions can fail if there is no support from the board and senior leadership when it comes down to the moment that decisions are made whether to tolerate a disruptive behavior or suffer a major financial loss.

The cost of a program to address behavioral issues pales in comparison to the damage. Collegial interactive teams are the foundation of patient safety (Nance, 2009). When a professional who has a history of disruptive behavior arrives on the unit, our attention is diverted away from critical responsibilities as we immediately begin monitoring their behavior for potential outbursts (Felps). Another study in the *Harvard Business Review* found that simply witnessing rude behavior has a significant affect on our ability to perform cognitive tasks (Porath). **Addressing disruptive behavior is our ethical**

obligation. "First do no harm" wasn't a suggestion. It is a moral imperative. "Disruptive behavior undermines practice morale, increases turnover, steals from other productive activities, increases risks for substandard practice, and distresses colleagues" (Bujak).

The investment in holding all staff accountable to the same standard of behavior pales in comparison to the return from that investment. Addressing conflict in the workplace yields multiple important cost-saving benefits, which are hard-wired firmly into the system for long run (Hickson):

- Improved staff satisfaction and retention

- Enhanced reputation for the medical center and its leaders

- Creation of a culture of professionals who are important role models for students, residents, staff, and each other

- Improved patient safety attributable to greater staff willingness to speak up when they observe patient care problems

- Reduced liability exposure and risk management activity

- Overall more productive, civil, and desirable work environments (Hickson)

Start Here: Roadmap to Success

Board and senior leadership commitment
"The ultimate responsibility for dealing with disruptive physicians rests with the governing board" (Bujak), and not a single medical director or CEO. Responsibility for enforcing behavioral standards should never be left to hospital administration. Ideally, evaluation

and enforcement is delegated to the credentialing committee of the medical staff. When this group has to choose between acting and doing the right thing or deferring the decision to the board, they will usually step up to the task at hand rather than allow an outside group to make the decision (Bujak).

Commitment from the senior leadership team needs to include a commitment to providing the education, time, finances, and other resources needed to create a policy, educate staff, and monitor a reporting system, as well as provide the feedback and emotional support required to champion a culture of collaboration.

One chief nurse stated, "I have a policy. We enforce it, but things haven't changed." In this institution, disruptive behavior was tolerated for years. Nurses had stopped reporting events because nothing was ever done. Furthermore, virtually no feedback was given to the individuals who did take the time to write up an incident report and use the new reporting system. Feedback is critical. Although senior leadership cannot share the details of a conversation, they most certainly can call the reporter of the event and say, "Thank you for taking the time to let us know about this. I want you to know that I've spoken with the physician. If anything like this ever happens again, or if you experience any retaliation, please call me directly."

Roadmap to Success

- Establish board and senior leadership commitment

- Set a standard of behavior/code of conduct

- Educate staff about the standard

- Integrate the code into the hospital culture

- Create a reporting or surveillance process

- Invest in system improvement

Source: Gerardi.

 Speak Your Truth

Set a standard of behavior/code of conduct

There's no need to reinvent a code from scratch. Professional behavior doesn't depend on what hospital you are working in, and many institutions are more than willing to share their behavioral policy (e.g., Vanderbilt Professional Conduct Policy) so that it becomes the standard across our professions.

A good policy will explicitly convey expectations, establish the correct reporting lines, and demonstrate the vision of healthy, collaborative relationships as set forth by senior leadership. Expectations should not only state the behaviors that are disruptive, but also the behaviors that are desirable. Most importantly, a code of conduct must be universal across the organization and aimed at ensuring high quality/safe care for patients (Gerardi).

> *"We wrote him up because he had egregiously violated not only our behavioral code, but the mission and values of our institution by cursing. But when they found out who it was, suddenly the whole incident just vanished into thin air as if it never happened at all. If his name wasn't on the report, or if he was a nurse, he'd be fired immediately."*
>
> *—ICU nurse*

Code of Conduct: Education and Integration

> *"System integration means processes designed to fit within the culture of the organization by those who will use them. These processes should allow flexible, emergent solutions to address complexity and facilitate learning" (Gerardi).*

An effective code or standard will contain a list of desirable behaviors:

- Identify and report quality concerns

- Give clear instructions for patient care

- Respectfully discuss concerns in a private setting

- Cooperate and participate in quality improvement activities

- Adhere to medical center bylaws and policies and procedures (Weber)

The code of conduct must explicitly define unprofessional behaviors:

- Demeaning behavior to staff or colleagues

- Inappropriate displays of anger or berating individuals

- Profane or disrespectful language or comments

- Condescending tone of voice in discussions or when answering questions

- Intimidating behavior that has the effect of suppressing necessary patient care communication or actions (Weber)

In other words, any behavior that makes you feel less than the competent, caring professional you are and that inhibits your desire and ability to speak your truth at any time is a disruptive behavior. Any behavior that impedes your ability to participate fully as a collegial team member. These include both overt and covert gestures and remarks, such as eye rolling, sighing, and lack of eye contact, as well as a lack of teamwork and ignoring a team member.

The code must clearly spell out behaviors that are considered disruptive and that will not be tolerated, such as:

- Criticizing staff or care in front of patients or families

- Throwing instruments, charts, or equipment

- Sexual comments or innuendos

- Unethical, illegal, or dishonest behavior

- Inappropriate comments in patient records or charting (Weber)

See Figure 4 for a continuum of professional behaviors.

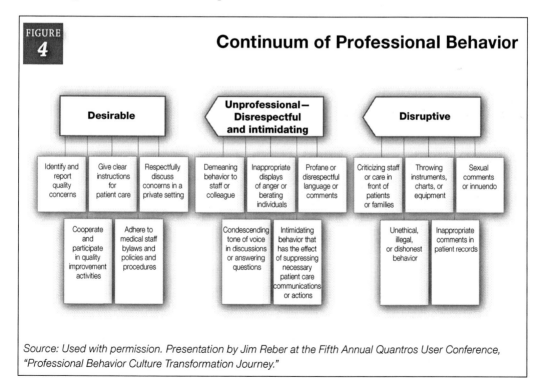

FIGURE 4

Continuum of Professional Behavior

Desirable

Identify and report quality concerns	Give clear instructions for patient care	Respectfully discuss concerns in a private setting

Cooperate and participate in quality improvement activities	Adhere to medical staff bylaws and policies and procedures

Unprofessional— Disrespectful and intimidating

Demeaning behavior to staff or colleague	Inappropriate displays of anger or berating individuals	Profane or disrespectful language or comments

Condescending tone of voice in discussions or answering questions	Intimidating behavior that has the effect of suppressing necessary patient care communications or actions

Disruptive

Criticizing staff or care in front of patients or families	Throwing instruments, charts, or equipment	Sexual comments or innuendo

Unethical, illegal, or dishonest behavior	Inappropriate comments in patient records

Source: Used with permission. Presentation by Jim Reber at the Fifth Annual Quantros User Conference, "Professional Behavior Culture Transformation Journey."

Different rules for different roles will never produce the desired outcomes. Many organizations continue to have separate expectations, education, and interventions depending on whether the individual is a physician or a nurse; a part of the medical staff or a hospital employee. Even if someone is not an employee of a hospital, if they have the privilege of walking through the doors, then the same rules apply to all. "Promoting professional conduct is not possible without leadership's commitment to addressing unprofessional/disruptive behaviors whenever they occur, regardless of the rank, or title of the physician who behaved poorly" (Hickson).

From theory to practice

As chief medical officer of St. Rita's Hospital, Dr. Herb Schumm, created and organized a "Coffee Corp" as a positive structured process for physicians to hold each other accountable for professional behaviors. He began by asking all physicians to write down the name of the physician for whom they had the most respect on an index card; then they turned the card over and wrote down the name of the physician who they believed would most likely be approached first when the new standards for professional behavior went into effect. (It was a surprise when a few physicians' names appeared on both sides of the card.) Six physicians stood out among the others as consistently respected by their peers. Schumm asked if they would attend a training course to increase their confidence and comfort level when following up on concerns with their peers.

After the training, "Coffee Corp" physicians would meet as needed with their peers on the platform of genuine concern. The meeting, which was informal and not scheduled, started with a collegial discussion of the concern to assess awareness of the issue and to ask why the behavior might have happened (awareness intervention). As is often the case, physicians were usually unaware of the effect their behavior had on others and, frequently, this single intervention was all that was needed.

After a code of conduct or behavioral standards is created and championed by leadership, a broad-based educational plan to disseminate the information to every group must then be implemented, followed by system integration (see Figure 5). Linking education to the core values of the institution is critical and shows employees that you are walking the talk. Integration of a conduct code requires hard-wiring the code into the hospital by including it in the faculty and employee handbook, medical staff bylaws, and practice group partnership agreements.

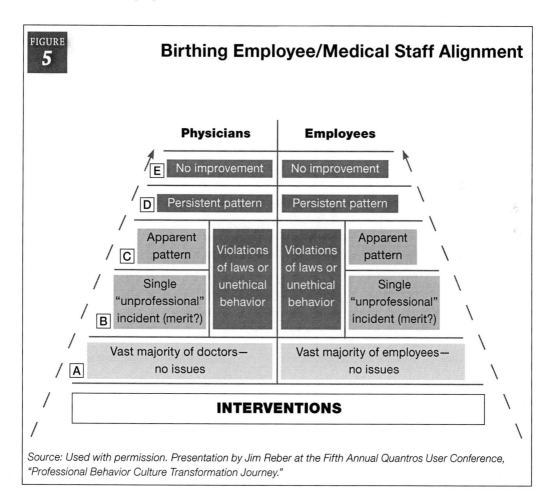

FIGURE 5

Birthing Employee/Medical Staff Alignment

Physicians			Employees	
E	No improvement		No improvement	
D	Persistent pattern		Persistent pattern	
C	Apparent pattern	Violations of laws or unethical behavior	Violations of laws or unethical behavior	Apparent pattern
B	Single "unprofessional" incident (merit?)			Single "unprofessional" incident (merit?)
A	Vast majority of doctors— no issues		Vast majority of employees— no issues	

INTERVENTIONS

Source: Used with permission. Presentation by Jim Reber at the Fifth Annual Quantros User Conference, "Professional Behavior Culture Transformation Journey."

Create a Reporting or Surveillance Process

"A standardized approach to reporting enables organizations to avoid many of the pit-
falls and inconsistencies that hamper the current processes" (Rosenstein). While the
best reporting systems are the eyes and ears of patients, family members, and employees,
studies show these people are hesitant to speak up or report problems (Hickson). Vanderbilt Medical Center addresses this fear by providing an inpatient video that encourages communication and feedback "so that we can attempt to make it right, as well as to
address and reduce the chance that others will experience the same outcome." Protecting
others from the same outcome is a stronger motivator than just speaking up for oneself.
Actively seeking feedback sends a strong message that you truly want the information
from patients and employees.

Structures and processes for reporting include setting up an electronic database, comment box, or phone hotline for complaints or hiring a patient advocate who can alert
leadership about incidents that warrant special attention (Hickson).

Nurses fear reporting MD-RN events because the incident is associated with feelings
of shame. In my experience, however, charge nurses always know about these events—
and often managers know as well—but the prevailing culture is a "don't rock the boat"
mentality. Reporting will only increase when staff members see that leadership means
what they say, demonstrated by taking action. The main blockade to nurse reporting is
the decades-old perception of "Why bother? Nothing ever changes."

But receiving reports is only half the work. It's what you do with the data that is critical.
Which group in your organization will be responsible for collecting and analyzing the data
so you have a heads up as to which units are experiencing a larger volume of complaints?

Invest in System Change

Senior leadership at St. Rita's perceived they were doing well managing disruptive behavior. From 2002 to 2007, they held 36 collegial interventions, six mandatory counseling sessions, four reprimands, and three suspensions. One physician moved across town to another hospital, and the others modified their behavior. But after a key incident with a senior physician, leadership took a second look. Maybe their perceptions weren't as accurate as they thought? Focusing on patient safety proved to be the game changer.

Leadership began by assessing the effect of disruptive behavior (DB) on daily care in four areas:

1. Perception of DB on patient care

2. Effectiveness of handling DB

3. Frequency of DB

4. Effect of DB

After analysis of the survey results, people using a condescending tone of voice scored the highest, and not just from physicians. Management discovered that staff avoided calling physicians and felt pressured to accept/execute an order in spite of their concerns. Survey results revealed a different reality from what leadership expected, which lead them to commit to transforming to a professional culture.

New language for addressing unprofessional or disruptive behavior was created, birthing a common language (Professional Behavior Continuum, Figure 4). The code of conduct was revised, and medical staff and HR tools were aligned. Interventions included positive reinforcement for the majority of physicians who were collegial and collaborative and interventions for unprofessional behavior that followed Hickson's pyramid model. Physicians were advised that St. Rita's had a zero-tolerance policy for overt or subtle retaliation. Transparency and disclosure became the new norms

---

Invest in System Change (cont.)

as interventions were shared with the employees involved in the events and timeout language was created for staff to use if they felt an event was escalating.

The effectiveness of the program and staff's perceptions were surveyed frequently. At the end of two years, St. Rita's witnessed phenomenal results. But it didn't stop there. Because of its ongoing commitment to patient safety, a plan for the following year (2009) was created to integrate TeamSTEPPS into the professional behaviors and the professional behaviors into the culture of safety initiative.

"Eliminating unprofessional behavior is an essential step to achieve authentic team-based care. With hindsight, the process seems remarkably similar to sexual harassment initiatives of the '90s," says CEO Jim Reber.

Cultural change such as this takes a strong, dedicated medical staff executive committee and senior leadership supported by the board. Any structure that encourages nurses and physicians to spend time together is a forcing function for improving healthy relationships: multidisciplinary rounds, intentional unit rounding, conflict management education, formalized communication models, joint educational events, RN-MD summits, interdisciplinary pathways, post-incident debriefing, etc. But the key is senior leadership commitment and a zero-tolerance policy. As Dr. Hickson says, "It's the right thing to do."

The Rest of the Bell Curve

The majority of this chapter has been spent addressing the less than 5% of physician behavior that is disruptive, as this is what healthcare leaders report takes up a considerable amount of their time, resources, and energy.

Now we can look at the other 95% and develop initiatives that support these physicians and the 10%–15% of whom are early adopters of collegial interactions. In order for our patients to be safe, the "friendly stranger" and "teacher-student" relationships must also improve significantly, for these account for a vast percentage of our relationships. What structures can organizations put in place to encourage and nurture collaborative nurse-physician relationships? Any process, system, or procedure that cuts across hierarchical boundaries is a winner.

Increase social capital

"Think of a king. In order for collegiality to ever happen, the king must take off his crown, AND the vassal must pick up her robe. Both robe and crown are symbols of power. To do either requires courage."

The easiest way to break across hierarchical/power boundaries is simply by getting to know each other as human beings, separate from our work roles. As it turns out, however, it's not that simple. Time and budget constraints, role identity, power, and the constant pressure for both groups to be more efficient are huge impediments to this end. There is a misperception in society (reflected in the medical community) that knowledge equals power.

One physician recently told me, "I don't like to go to the quality meetings with the nurses because I always end up feeling emasculated." This comment reflects an often-held belief that to collaborate means giving away power. To him, the experience of working outside his physician role was perceived as a weakness (to work with the vassals instead of fellow kings). To expose himself as a human being who is fallible and needs the help of his team members is uncomfortable to say the least—just as uncomfortable as it is for nurses to use SBAR and actually make a recommendation. (As uncomfortable as it would be for a vassal to give advice to a king, fearing the words "Off with his/her head!) Connecting as human beings holds infinite rewards for us all.

Time is a precious commodity, and even if we create the physical spaces, both physicians and nurses are working 12-hour shifts and are tired. When was the last time something fun happened in your department or hospital? Celebration is a characteristic of a healthy work community, and administration is in the perfect position to sponsor a joint event annually.

It's critical to have key staff members weave between the two groups and bridge the hierarchy or to use a tool that fosters connection. An example mentioned earlier in the book is to create name tags that list a favorite hobby or vacation spot; another is to hold a Truth or Dare section of a meeting so people can get to know each other. Social capital, the energy formed by relationships, is as vital as financial capital (Putnam). Our greatest strength is in each other. **What event could you sponsor that would act as a forcing function to propel traditional nurse-physician relationships deeper than the mask of composure?** In our three-month orientation, nurses now spend an entire day following a physician, even if he has surgery. Sharing a day's work and a meal has been a wonderful forcing function. Physicians appear to have more vested interest in the new staff and new nurses do not hesitate as much to approach a physician.

As well as connecting on a human level, there are system changes that can be made to enhance communication. Standardized protocols "reduce the need for nurses to call physicians and help manage patient care more efficiently" (Sirota). Protocols decrease the frequency of unnecessary calls while at the same time increasing the sense of autonomy among nursing professionals who are encouraged to use their clinical assessment skills and judgment. The very process of creating protocols increases collaboration because this work promotes cooperation, interaction, and most importantly, education about the different yet overlapping roles of nurses and physicians.

There is no longer any debating that standardization of such items as protocols and checklists prevents harm. Avoidable mistakes "continue to plague health care ... because the volume and complexity of knowledge today has exceeded our capacity as individuals to properly deliver it to people—consistently, correctly, safely" (Gawande). However, leaders still report that physicians hesitate to use these life-saving tools because it threatens the core value of their profession: autonomy. Gawande's book, *A Checklist Manifesto,* is an excellent resource for physician transformation in this area.

There is no debating that healthcare organizations are high-reliability organizations (HRO), as they are places where human life is at stake and stress and potential for error are high. Other examples of HROs include nuclear power plants and infectious disease control. Proven best practice from HROs for improved communication include using structured language, which is proven to consistently ensure clear and concise communication and reduce errors. One technique is SBAR, which is described in detail in Chapter 5. A study using SBAR improved nurses' perception of their ability to communicate effectively with physicians in their daily interactions about patient care. Having a systematic approach turned out to be an important component of self-efficacy. Even using the tool in a role-playing situation, however, nurses were reluctant to communicate assertively with rude or disruptive physicians (Raica). Using SBAR in a simulation can be extremely beneficial, especially as a post-debriefing following communication failures.

One of the major hurdles with SBAR, or other structured communication models, has been that nurses are educated in the model, but physicians are not. Nurses then report feeling sabotaged when they use the model, make a recommendation, and are shut down by physicians. Likewise, physicians are equally caught off guard to hear nurses suggest a course of action. This model pushes people beyond their comfort zone, so education must always include both groups.

Another communication model is STICC, which fosters understanding between parties so that failures are averted. The advantage to this model is that it requires feedback, thereby inviting two-way communication. The model is as follows:

S – Situation	"Here's what I think we face."
T – Task	"Here's what I think we should do."
I – Intent	"Here's why …"
C – Concern	"Here's what we should keep our eye on."
C – Calibrate	"Now talk to me: Tell me if you don't understand, cannot do it, or see something that I don't (Sutcliffe et al.)."

Increase nurse educational level

Another way to improve communication is to even the education playing field. Work with local colleges to provide nurses with easy access to education, and establish a scholarship or reimbursement program to encourage nurses to pursue higher education. You can provide easy access to education through online courses.

Encourage all nurses in leadership roles, especially charge nurses, to attain advanced degrees, and set a hiring preference/requirement for nurses with a BSN degree. Encourage or sponsor a speaker to come to your hospital and prepare nurses for national certification in their specialty as this also contributes to clinical competence. Significant differences have been found between perceptions of empowerment and intent to leave a current position between certified and non-certified nurses (*American Journal of Critical Care*, 2010). One acute care medical unit in a 750-bed Virginia hospital increased the percentage of certified nurses by 60% in one year, which lead to increases in RN satisfaction in the areas of teamwork, participation in unit-based decision making, and professional development. All these are indicative of increased empowerment and engagement (*MedSurg Nursing*, 2007).

Monitor the number of BSN-educated nurses on a unit and organizational level and set target dates and target percentages for numbers of nurses who will have BSNs. "Competent performance and self confidence are the keys to both collaborative nurse-physician relationships and clinical autonomy" (Schmalenberg). Physicians' perception of nurses as lacking competence was the major factor behind low ratings when physicians were asked to score the degree of interdisciplinary collaboration (Schmalenberg). While competence is linked to both experience and education, self-esteem, self-confidence, increased knowledge, and self-efficacy increase as we ascend the educational ladder.

Seek ANCC Magnet Recognition Program® status

Another method for improving relationships is to seek ANCC Magnet Recognition Program® (MRP) designation. Compared to non-designated hospitals, nurses in MRP hospitals consistently report higher-quality nurse-physician relationships (Schmalenberg, Kramer, 2009). The climate of relationships is 80% collegial and collaborative, with the next most prominent relationship group being student-teacher. This reflects the fact that nursing autonomy is higher in MRP hospitals because the essence of the structure promotes nurses having a voice through shared governance.

Conflict resolution skills

Even MRP hospitals have experienced a trend of increasing adversarial relationships from 11% in 2001 to 17% in 2007 (Schmalenberg, Kramer). This trend no doubt parallels the increased pressures that both doctors and nurses feel coming from all sides: legal, moral, financial, time constraints, technology, etc. Add these pressures to a group of physicians and nurses who avoid conflict at any cost, and the reasons for mandating education to improve our confrontation skills becomes apparent.

The Joint Commission expects organizations to manage conflict between leadership groups so that the quality and safety of care is protected (LD 2.40). According to this standard, the conflict process must include meeting with the involved parties as early as possible to identify conflict, gathering information, and working with the parties to address and resolve the conflict if possible. Individuals who implement the process must be skilled in conflict management, which, as discussed earlier, is lacking for both physicians and nurses.

In addition, the goal is to have all conflict resolved at the unit level. This can only happen if staff are given a tool set to engage in the confrontation and have manager backup. It is critical that hospital leadership commit to an education program that gives all employees the skills to manage confrontations effectively and professionally and that hardwires this education into the organization. The key to cultural change is for leaders to consistently focus on behavior and language (Logan). **Manager support is the most frequently cited structure by nurses and physicians as a contributing factor to collegial relationships** (Schmalenberg, 2005).

Hold the Vision

"Articulating [a] positive vision is the primary responsibility of leadership" (Bujak). Every nurse and physician leader who has a vision paints a picture of a place that no one has ever seen before. They paint this picture every day by their words and actions. Some paintings are larger than life and easily seen by all; others are tiny miniatures depending on our level of awareness and commitment. We paint these visions with our passion and commitment for improved nurse-physician relationships.

What would it look like if nurses and physicians were truly collegial partners who couldn't imagine patient care without each other? Colleagues who constantly invited each other's insights, feedback, and thoughts; who understood how vital they are to each other and enjoyed each other's company by sharing life stories, coffee, or even the same dining room? What if medical apartheid no longer existed? If the respect and trust level between nurses and physicians was such that communication was seamless and the boundaries of roles and power long forgotten? Not only would our relationships with each other nurture and sustain us, but our patients, who entrust themselves to our care, would be safe.

"People embrace a vision not for what it says, but for what it does, not because it is probable, but rather because it is irresistible."

J. Bujak, MD

References

Buerhaus, P.I., K. Donelan, B.T. Ulrich, I. Norman, M. Williams, and R. Dittus. (2005). "Hospital RN's and CNO's Perceptions of the Impact of the Nursing Shortage on the Quality of Care." *Nursing Economic$* 23(5): 214–21, 211.

Bujak, J.S. (2008) *Inside the Physician Mind: Finding Common Ground With Doctors.* Chicago: Health Administration Press.

Craven, H. (2007). "Recognizing Excellence: Unit-based Activities to Support Specialty Nursing Certification." *MedSur Nursing* 16 (6).

Eddy, W.A. (2003) *High Conflict Personalities: Understanding and Resolving Their Costly Disputes.* San Diego: William Eddy.

Eddy, W.A. (2008) *It's All Your Fault! Twelve Tips for Managing People Who Blame Others for Everything.* Calgary, Canada: Janis Publications.

Felps, W., T.R. Mitchell, and E. Byington. (2006). "How, When and Why Bad Apples Spoil the Barrel: Negative Group Members and Dysfunctional Groups." *Research in Organizational Behavior: An Annual Series of Analytical Essays and Critical Reviews* 27: 175–222.

Fitzpatrick, J., T.M. Campo, G. Graham, and R. Lavandero. (2010). "Certification, Empowerment, and Intent to Leave Current Position and the Profession Among Critical Care Nurses." *American Journal of Critical Care.* Gawande, A. *(2009). The Checklist Manifesto: How to Get Things Right.* New York: Metropolitan Books/Henry Holt and Co.

Gerardi, D. (2008). "Creating Cultures of Engagement: Effective Strategies for Addressing Conflict and 'Disruptive' Behavior." PowerPoint presentation.

Gerardi, D., and D.K. Fontaine. (2007). "True Collaboration: Envisioning New Ways of Working Together." *AACN Advanced Critical Care* 18 (1): 10–14.

Gerardi, D. (2007). "The Emerging Culture of Health Care: Improving End-of-Life Care Through Collaboration and Conflict Engagement Among Health Care Professionals." *Ohio State Journal on Dispute Resolution* 23 (1).

Hickson, G.B, Pichert, J.W., Webb, L.E., and Gabbe, S.G. (2007). "A complementary approach to promoting professionalism: Identifying, measuring, and addressing unprofessional behaviors." *Academic Medicine* 82 (11): 1040–1048.

The Joint Commission. (2008). "Behaviors That Undermine a Culture of Safety." *www.jointcommission.org/ NewsRoom/PressKits/Behaviors+that+Undermine+a+Culture+of+Safety/app_stds.htm* (accessed August 2008).

Logan, D., J. King, and H. Fischer-Wright. (2008). "Tribal leadership: Leveraging Natural Groups to Build a Thriving Organization. New York: Harper Business.

Nance, John (2009). *Why Hospitals Should Fly.* Bozeman, MT: Second River Healthcare.

National Joint Practice Commission. (1974). *Guidelines for Establishing Joint or Collaborative Practice in Hospitals.* Chicago: Nealy Printing.

Porath, C, and A. Erez. "Does Rudeness Really Matter? The Effects of Rudeness on Task Performance and Helpfulness." *Academy of Management Journal* 50 (5): 1181–1197.

Raica, D. (2009). "Effect of Action-Oriented Communication Training on Nurses' Communication Self-Efficacy." *Med Surg Nursing* 18 (6).

Schmalenberg, C., and M. Kramer. (2009). "Nurse-Physician Relationships in Hospitals: 20,000 Nurses Tell Their Story." *Critical Care Nurse* 29 (1).

Sirota, T. (2007). "Nurse-Physician Relationships: Improving or Not?" *Nursing* 37 (1).

Sutcliffe, K.M., E. Lewton, and M.M. Rosenthal. (2004). "Communication Failures: An Insidious Contributor to Medical Mishaps." *Academic Medicine* 79 (2): 186–194.

The Washington Post. (2007). "Pearls Before Breakfast: Can One of the Nation's Great Musicians Cut Through the Fog of a D.C. Rush Hour? Let's Find Out." *www.washingtonpost.com/wp-dyn/content/article/2007/04/04/AR2007040401721.html?hpid=topnews* (accessed March 17, 2010).

Weber, David O. (2004). "Poll Results: Doctors' Disruptive Behavior Disturbs Physician Leaders." *The Physician Executive* 30 (4): 6–14.

Continuing Education Credits

Continuing education credits are available for this book for two years from date of purchase.

Target Audience

Staff nurses, charge nurses, nurse managers, preceptors, clinical nurse leaders, staff development professionals, directors of staff development, directors of nursing, VPs of nursing, chief nursing officers, chief nurse executives, VPs of patient care services.

Statement of Need

This book approaches nurse-physician communication trouble spots by coupling anecdotal scenarios with tangible advice for nurses. It offers field-tested, how-to advice for helping nurses fully understand and cope with communication breakdowns that often occur between doctors and nurses. The book includes case scenarios, critical-thinking activities, and other tools to help nurses better understand and communicate with physicians. It also includes advice for leadership about creating and sustaining healthy work environments. (This activity is intended for individual use only.)

Educational Objectives

Upon completion of this activity, participants should be able to:

- Define the "chain of command" infrastructure, where it began, and when it should be activated in the hospital setting

- Explain passive-aggressive communication and give one specific example of this communication from your work setting in nursing

- Explain the key concept in "Crew Resource Management" and how this philosophy applies to healthcare

- State the oppression theory and explain its application to physician-nurse relationships

- Identify two common learned behaviors physicians employ when interacting with nurses

- Recognize and explain the roots of the subordinate role of the nurse

- Identify the key stakeholders and how their relationships affect each other

- Relate the occurrence of sentinel events to non- or miscommunication among physicians and nurses

- Define "horizontal violence" and identify two specific examples in your current work setting

- List and explain the five categories of relationship that help define nurse-physician relationships

- State two possible follow-up actions nurses can take to facilitate communication within each category of nurse-physician relationships

- List key steps used for calling difficult physicians on the telephone

- Explain how administrative support, a zero-tolerance policy, and assertiveness training are used as opportunities for improving nurse-physician relationships

- List and describe two practical strategies for nurturing relationships on your unit

- List the conversation tips for confronting a disruptive physician about his behavior

- List two actions that nurse managers should take to combat disruptive behavior

- Describe leadership's role in creating and sustaining healthy nurse-physician relationships

- Discuss strategies leaders can use to deal with disruptive behavior

Faculty

Kathleen Bartholomew, RN, MN, managed a 57-bed orthopedic and spine unit in a tertiary hospital in Seattle for five years before turning to writing and public speaking full time. The first edition of *Speak Your Truth* was accepted as her master's thesis while studying at the University of Washington, Bothell.

Continuing Education

Nursing Contact Hours:

HCPro, Inc., is accredited as a provider of continuing nursing education by the American Nurses Credentialing Center Commission on Accreditation.

This educational activity for 3.5 nursing contact hours is provided by HCPro, Inc.

Faculty Disclosure Statement

HCPro, Inc., has confirmed that none of the faculty, contributors, or planners have any relevant financial relationships to disclose related to the content of this educational activity.

Disclosure of Unlabeled Use

This educational activity may contain discussion of published and/or investigational uses of agents that are not indicated by the FDA. HCPro, Inc., does not recommend the use of any agent outside of the labeled indications. The opinions expressed in the educational activity are those of the faculty and do not necessarily represent the views of HCPro, Inc. Please refer to the official prescribing information for each product for discussion of approved indications, contraindications, and warnings.

Instructions

In order to be eligible to receive your nursing contact hours for this activity, you are required to do the following:

1. Read the book *Speak Your Truth: Proven Strategies for Effective Nurse-Physician Communication*

2. Complete the exam and receive a passing score of 80%

3. Complete the evaluation

4. Provide your contact information on the exam and evaluation

5. Submit exam and evaluation to HCPro, Inc.

Please provide all of the information requested above and mail or fax your completed exam, program evaluation, and contact information to

> HCPro, Inc.
> Attention: Continuing Education Manager
> P.O. Box 1168
> Marblehead, MA 01945
> Fax: 781/639-2982

Note:

This book and associated exam are intended for individual use only. If you would like to provide this continuing education exam to other members of your nursing or physician staff, please contact our customer service department at 877/727-1728 to place your order. The exam fee schedule is as follows:

Exam Quantity	Fee
1	$0
2 – 25	$15 per person
26 – 50	$12 per person
51 – 100	$8 per person
101+	$5 per person

Continuing Education Exam

Name: _____

Title: _____

Facility name: _____

Address: _____

Address: _____

City: _____ State: _____ ZIP: _____

Phone number: _____ Fax number: _____

E-mail: _____

Date completed: _____

1. **According to the text, the current nursing infrastructure robs the nurse of his or her autonomy. What is this system called?**

    a. Oppression theory

    b. Chain of command

    c. Aunt Jane

    d. Good Samaritan

2. **Doctor: "Nurse, you were completely out of line by questioning my plan of care for the patient. Next time you have a suggestion, keep it to yourself!"**

    Nurse: "Fine." The nurse later reenacts the scene for her nurse colleagues. She says nothing to the doctor about his behavior and will continue to carry a grudge for years to come.

    What form of behavior is the nurse demonstrating?

    a. Assertion

    b. Dominance

    c. Confrontational

    d. Passive-aggression

 Speak Your Truth

3. The "Crew Resource Management" philosophy states that every member of a team has a responsibility to speak up when in doubt, to confirm and question orders, and to offer insight. Further, the commander has a responsibility to create and nurture this type of environment. This philosophy's importance to healthcare is underlined by the Institute of Medicine's 1999 report, which estimated that _____ people die every year from medical errors.

    a. 1,000–48,000

    b. 48,000–98,000

    c. 98,000–148,000

    d. 148,000–198,000

4. According to the oppression theory, when there is a dominant group there must also be a subordinate group. The book refers to physicians as the dominant group and nurses as the subordinate group. Which group is responsible for this inequality, which continues between nurses and physicians?

    a. Nurses are responsible for perpetuating inequality

    b. Physicians are responsible for perpetuating inequality

    c. Both nurses and physicians are responsible for perpetuating inequality

    d. Patients are responsible for perpetuating inequality

5. A negative tone of voice, no eye contact, and not calling nurses by their names are all _____ by physicians.

    a. communication techniques

    b. learned behaviors

    c. passive-aggressive behaviors

    d. teaching techniques

6. The _____ model teaches separation, dissection, and objective and linear thinking and has a heavy influence on medicine.

    a. Western medical

    b. caring

    c. Florence Nightingale

    d. subjective-holistic

7. In order to improve nurse-physician relationships significantly, we must understand the roles of key stakeholders. In the text, who are the four key stakeholders?

    a. Provider, nurse, physician, and charge nurse

    b. Provider, nurse, physician, and nurse manager

    c. Patient, family, nurse, and physician

    d. Patient, nurse, physician, and nurse manager

8. The root cause of 2,455 sentinel events analyzed by The Joint Commission found that 70% of the cases were due to communication failure. What percentage of these patients died?

    a. 25%

    b. 50%

    c. 75%

    d. 100%

9. When members of an oppressed group lash out against each other either openly or with passive-aggression, this is known as _____.

    a. assertion

    b. dominance

    c. horizontal violence

    d. vertical violence

 Speak Your Truth

10. There are five relationship categories used to describe the state of nurse-physician relationships. These categories include collegial, collaborative, teacher-student, friendly stranger, and hostile. Out of the five, which relationship produces positive outcomes for patients, leaves the nurse feeling less powerful, and always allows the physician the last word?

    a. Collegial

    b. Collaborative

    c. Teacher-student

    d. Friendly stranger

    e. Hostile

11. Within the text, the author instructs readers to first establish a relationship with physicians by using humor, social events, or conversation to bring physicians out of their shell. To what category of relationship is she offering follow-up advice?

    a. Collegial

    b. Collaborative

    c. Teacher-student

    d. Friendly stranger

    e. Hostile

12. When placing a call to a physician, there are certain actions you can take to be sure that the call goes smoothly. From the list below, choose the answer that best illustrates the incorrect way to speak to a physician.

    a. Don't begin with an apology. Begin with identifying yourself and the patient.

    b. Always have the chart, labs, and latest vital signs in hand.

    c. Repeat back to the physician a summary of the order or the conversation.

    d. Take your time; slowly, with narration, explain what you need.

13. _____ techniques recommend using short, specific statements that describe the event or behavior, such as, "Please do not yell. If you continue to yell I will leave," or, "I did not appreciate the comments you made in front of the patient today."

    a. Administrative support

    b. Assertiveness training

    c. Zero-tolerance policy

    d. SBAR model

14. **What does SBAR stand for?**

    a. Situation, Background, Assessment, Recommendation

    b. Situation, Background, Assertion, Reconciliation

    c. Situation, Background, Assumption, Recommendation

    d. Situation, Background, Assistance, Reconciliation

15. **Finding a private place (e.g., a conference room) where you can sit down, always taking potentially emotional conversations off the floor, making excellent eye contact, and being direct are all tips listed to help nurses handle conversations with _____.**

    a. personal acquaintances

    b. fellow nurses

    c. sick patients

    d. disruptive physicians

16. **To facilitate healthy nurse-physician relationships, nurse managers should _____.**

    a. stay out of nurse-physician relationships

    b. keep separate educational events for nurses and physicians

    c. insist that physicians call staff by name

    d. help nurses get back at disruptive physicians

17. The text refers to a survey of 1,627 physician executives about disruptive behaviors. What percentage of respondents indicated their organization had a code of conduct in place?

    a. 11%

    b. 51%

    c. 61%

    d. 71%

18. Which of the following is NOT a reason why medical directors have difficulty handling peer behavioral issues?

    a. They can't suspend or fire colleagues

    b. They are unprepared to handle conflict

    c. They do not want to break a cultural code

    d. They support unprofessional behavior

19. According to Hickson et al.'s model, which of the following is an appropriate response to a single unprofessional incident?

    a. Cup of coffee conversation

    b. Awareness intervention

    c. Authority intervention

    d. Disciplinary intervention

20. Which of the following is an appropriate response to a pattern of unprofessional behavior?

    a. Cup of coffee conversation

    b. Awareness intervention

    c. Authority intervention

    d. Disciplinary intervention

Continuing Education Exam Answer Key

(Please record all exam and evaluation answers here)

Name: _____   License #: _____

Facility: _____   Title: _____

Address: _____

City: _____   State: _____   ZIP: _____

Phone: _____

E-mail: _____
(Certificates are e-mailed to learners unless otherwise stated here)

Please record the letter of the correct answer to the corresponding exam question below:				
1.	5.	9.	13.	17.
2.	6.	10.	14.	18.
3.	7.	11.	15.	19.
4.	8.	12.	16.	20.

Continuing Education Evaluation

1 = Strongly Agree   **2** = Agree   **3** = Disagree   **4** = Strongly Disagree

(Please rate the responses below according to the scale above to rate the quality of this educational activity)

1. **Please indicate how well you feel this activity met the learning objectives listed:**   1   2   3   4

2. **Objectives were related to the overall purpose/goal of the activity:**   1   2   3   4

3. **This activity was related to my continuing education needs:**   1   2   3   4

4. The exam for the activity was an accurate test of the
   knowledge gained: 1   2   3   4

5. The activity avoided commercial bias or influence: 1   2   3   4

6. This activity met my expectations: 1   2   3   4

7. The format was an appropriate method for delivery
   of the content for this activity: 1   2   3   4

8. Will this activity enhance your professional practice?
   Yes   No

9. How much time did it take for you to complete this activity?

   _____

10. Do you have any additional comments on this activity?

   _____

   _____

   _____

   _____

   _____

Return completed form to:

HCPro, Inc. • Attention: Continuing Education Manager • P.O. Box 1168, Marblehead, MA 01945

Telephone: 877/727-1728 • Fax: 781/639-2982

FREE HEALTHCARE COMPLIANCE AND MANAGEMENT RESOURCES!

Need to control expenses yet stay current with critical issues?

Get timely help with FREE e-mail newsletters from HCPro, Inc., the leader in healthcare compliance education. Offering numerous free electronic publications covering a wide variety of essential topics, you'll find just the right e-newsletter to help you stay current, informed, and effective. All you have to do is sign up!

With your FREE subscriptions, you'll also receive the following:

- Timely information, to be read when convenient with your schedule
- Expert analysis you can count on
- Focused and relevant commentary
- Tips to make your daily tasks easier

And here's the best part: There's no further obligation—just a complimentary resource to help you get through your daily challenges.

It's easy. Visit *www.hcmarketplace.com/free/e-newsletters* to register for as many free e-newsletters as you'd like, and let us do the rest.

$+$HCPro | Insight for healthcare compliance and management